Virtual Clinical Excursions—Obstetrics-Pediatrics

for

McKinney, James, Murray, and Ashwill:
Maternal-Child Nursing,
2nd Edition

Virtual Clinical Excursions—Obstetrics-Pediatrics

for

McKinney, James, Murray, and Ashwill:
Maternal-Child Nursing,
2nd Edition

prepared by

Kitty Cashion, RN, BC, MSN
Clinical Nurse Specialist
University of Tennessee, Memphis, Health Science Center
Department of Obstetrics and Gynecology
Division of Maternal-Fetal Medicine
Memphis, Tennessee

Kelly Ann Crum, RN, MSN
Instructional Specialist
Lead Faculty
Curriculum Development/Maternal Child Nursing Specialty
Health Sciences and Nursing Department
University of Phoenix, Online
Phoenix, Arizona

Betty W. Hamlisch, RN, MS Health Education
Professor of Nursing
Tompkins Cortland Community College
Dryden, New York

software developed by

Wolfsong Informatics, LLC
Tucson, Arizona

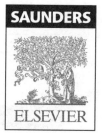

SAUNDERS

ELSEVIER

SAUNDERS
ELSEVIER

11830 Westline Industrial Dr.
St. Louis, Missouri 63146

VIRTUAL CLINICAL EXCURSIONS—OBSTETRICS-PEDIATRICS FOR
MCKINNEY, JAMES, MURRAY, AND ASHWILL:
MATERNAL-CHILD NURSING
SECOND EDITION
Copyright © 2006, Elsevier Inc.

ISBN 13: 978-1-4160-0104-1
ISBN 10: 1-4160-0104-2

Notice

Knowledge and best practice in this field are constantly changing. As new research and experience
broaden our knowledge, changes in practice, treatment and drug therapy may become necessary or
appropriate. Readers are advised to check the most current information provided (i) on procedures
featured or (ii) by the manufacturer of each product to be administered, to verify the recommended
dose or formula, the method and duration of administration, and contraindications. It is the
responsibility of the practitioner, relying on their own experience and knowledge of the patient, to
make diagnoses, to determine dosages and the best treatment for each individual patient, and to
take all appropriate safety precautions. To the fullest extent of the law, neither the Publisher nor
the Authors assumes any liability for any injury and/or damage to persons or property arising out
or related to any use of the material contained in this book.

ISBN 13: 978-1-4160-0104-1
ISBN 10: 1-4160-0104-2

Executive Editor, Nursing: *Tom Wilhelm*
Managing Editor: *Jeff Downing*
Associate Developmental Editor: *Jennifer Stoces*
Project Manager: *Joy Moore*

Printed in the United States of America

Last digit is the print number: 9 8 7 6 5 4 3 2

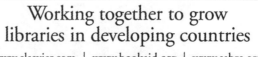

Working together to grow
libraries in developing countries

www.elsevier.com | www.bookaid.org | www.sabre.org

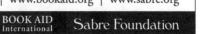

ELSEVIER   BOOK AID
International   Sabre Foundation

Workbook
prepared by

Kitty Cashion, RN, BC, MSN
Clinical Nurse Specialist
University of Tennessee, Memphis, Health Science Center
Department of Obstetrics and Gynecology
Division of Maternal-Fetal Medicine
Memphis, Tennessee

Kelly Ann Crum, RN, MSN
Instructional Specialist
Lead Faculty
Curriculum Development/Maternal Child Nursing Specialty
Health Sciences and Nursing Department
University of Phoenix, Online
Phoenix, Arizona

Betty W. Hamlisch, RN, MS Health Education
Professor of Nursing
Tompkins Cortland Community College
Dryden, New York

Textbook

Emily Slone McKinney, MSN, RN
Baylor University Medical Center
Women and Children's Services
Dallas, Texas

Susan Rowen James, MSN, RN
Associate Professor of Nursing
Division of Nursing Studies
Curry College
Milton, Massachusetts

Sharon Smith Murray, MSN, RN
Professor, Health Professions
Golden West College
Huntington Beach, California

Jean W. Ashwill, MSN, RN
Director of Undergraduate Student Services
School of Nursing
University of Texas, Arlington
Arlington, Texas

Contents

Table of Contents
McKinney, James, Murray, and Ashwill:
Maternal-Child Nursing, 2nd Edition

Pediatric Nursing Care

Appendixes

The following appendix can be found online at *http://evolve.elsevier.com/McKinney/mat-ch/*

Getting Started

GETTING SET UP

■ **MINIMUM SYSTEM REQUIREMENTS**

WINDOWS™

Windows XP, 2000, 98, ME, NT 4.0 (Recommend Windows XP/2000)
Pentium® III processor (or equivalent) @ 600 MHz (Recommend 800 MHz or better)
128 MB of RAM (Recommend 256 MB or more)
800 x 600 screen size (Recommend 1024 x 768)
Thousands of colors
12x CD-ROM drive
Soundblaster 16 soundcard compatibility
Stereo speakers or headphones

Note: Virtual Clinical Excursions—Obstetrics-Pediatrics for Windows will require a minimal amount of disk space to install icons and required dll files for Windows 98/ME.

MACINTOSH®

MAC OS X (10.2 or higher)
Apple Power PC G3 @ 500 MHz or better
128 MB of RAM (Recommend 256 MB or more)
800 x 600 screen size (Recommend 1024 x 768)
Thousands of colors
12x CD-ROM drive
Stereo speakers or headphones

1

■ INSTALLATION INSTRUCTIONS

WINDOWS

1. Insert the *Virtual Clinical Excursions—Obstetrics-Pediatrics* CD-ROM.
2. Inserting the CD should automatically bring up the setup screen if the current product is not already installed.
   a. If the setup screen does not appear automatically (and *Virtual Clinical Excursions— Obstetrics-Pediatrics* has not been installed already), navigate to the "My Computer" icon on your desktop or in your Start menu.
   b. Double-click on your CD-ROM drive.
   c. If installation does not start at this point:
      (1) Click the **Start** icon on the task bar and select the **Run** option.
      (2) Type d:\setup.exe (where "d:\" is your CD-ROM drive) and press **OK**.
      (3) Follow the onscreen instructions for installation.
3. Follow the onscreen instructions during the setup process.

MACINTOSH

1. Insert the *Virtual Clinical Excursions—Obstetrics-Pediatrics* CD in the CD-ROM drive. The disk icon will appear on your desktop.

2. Double-click on the disk icon.

3. Double-click on the VCEOBPE_MAC run file.

NOTE: *Virtual Clinical Excursions—Obstetrics-Pediatrics* for Macintosh does not have an installation setup and can only be run directly from the CD.

■ HOW TO USE VIRTUAL CLINICAL EXCURSIONS—OBSTETRICS-PEDIATRICS

WINDOWS

1. Double-click on the *Virtual Clinical Excursions—Obstetrics-Pediatrics* icon located on your desktop.
2. Or navigate to the program via the Windows Start menu.

NOTE: Windows 98/ME will require you to restart your computer before running the *Virtual Clinical Excursions—Obstetrics-Pediatrics* program.

MACINTOSH

1. Insert the *Virtual Clinical Excursions—Obstetrics-Pediatrics* CD in the CD-ROM drive. The disk icon will appear on your desktop.

2. Double-click on the disk icon.

3. Double-click on the VCEOBPE_MAC run file.

■ SCREEN SETTINGS

For best results, your computer monitor resolution should be set at a minimum of 800 x 600. The number of colors displayed should be set to "thousands or higher" (High Color or 16 bit) or "millions of colors" (True Color or 24 bit).

Windows™

1. From the **Start** menu, select **Control Panel** (on some systems, you will first go to **Settings**, then to **Control Panel**).
2. Double-click on the **Display** icon.
3. Click on the **Settings** tab.
4. Under **Screen area** use the slider bar to select **800 by 600 pixels**.
5. Access the **Colors** drop-down menu by clicking on the down arrow.
6. Select **High Color (16 bit)** or **True Color (24 bit)**.
7. Click on **OK**.
8. You may be asked to verify the setting changes. Click **Yes**.
9. You may be asked to restart your computer to accept the changes. Click **Yes**.

Macintosh®

1. Select the **Monitors** control panel.
2. Select **800 x 600** (or similar) from the **Resolution** area.
3. Select **Thousands** or **Millions** from the **Color Depth** area.

■ WEB BROWSERS

Supported web browsers include Microsoft Internet Explorer (IE) version 5.0 or higher and Netscape version 4.5 or higher. *Note that Netscape version 6.0 is not supported at this time, although versions 6.2 and higher are supported.*

If you use America Online (AOL) for web access, you will need AOL version 4.0 or higher and IE 5.0 or higher. Do not use earlier versions of AOL with earlier versions of IE, because you will have difficulty accessing many features.

For best results with AOL:
- Connect to the Internet using AOL version 4.0 or higher.
- Open a private chat within AOL (this allows the AOL client to remain open, without asking whether you wish to disconnect while minimized).
- Minimize AOL.
- Launch a recommended browser.

■ TECHNICAL SUPPORT

Technical support for this product is available between 7:30 a.m. and 7 p.m. CST, Monday through Friday. Before calling, be sure that your computer meets the minimum system requirements to run this software. Inside the United States and Canada, call 1-800-692-9010. Outside North America, call 314-872-8370. You may also fax your questions to 314-997-5080 or contact Technical Support through e-mail: technical.support@elsevier.com.

Trademarks: Windows, Macintosh, Pentium, and America Online are registered trademarks.

ACCESSING *Virtual Clinical Excursions—Obstetrics-Pediatrics* FROM EVOLVE ————————

The product you have purchased is part of the Evolve family of online courses and learning resources. Please read the following information completely to get started.

To access your instructor's course on Evolve:

Your instructor will provide you with the username and password needed to access their specific course on the Evolve Learning System. Once you have received this information, please follow these instructions:

1. Go to the Evolve student page (http://evolve.elsevier.com/student).

2. Enter your username and password in the **Login to My Evolve** area and click the **Login** button.

3. You will be taken to your personalized **My Evolve** page where the course will be listed in the **My Courses** module.

TECHNICAL REQUIREMENTS

To use an Evolve course, you will need access to a computer that is connected to the Internet and equipped with web browser software that supports frames. For optimal performance, it is recommended that you have speakers and use a high-speed Internet connection. However, slower dial-up modems (56 K minimum) are acceptable.

Whichever browser you use, the browser preferences must be set to enable cookies and Java/JavaScript and the cache must be set to reload every time.

<u>Enable Cookies</u>

Browser	Steps
Internet Explorer 5.0 or higher	1. Select **Tools**. 2. Select **Internet Options**. 3. Select **Security** tab. 4. Make sure **Internet** (globe) is highlighted. 5. Select **Custom Level** button. 6. Scroll down the **Security Settings** list. 7. Under **Cookies** heading, make sure **Enable** is selected. 8. Click **OK**.
Internet Explorer 6.0	1. Select **Tools**. 2. Select **Internet Options**. 3. Select **Privacy** tab. 4. Use the slider (slide down) to **Accept All Cookies**. 5. Click **OK**. -OR- 4. Click the **Advanced** button. 5. Click the check box next to **Override Automatic Cookie Handling**. 6. Click the **Accept** buttons under **First-party Cookies** and **Third-party Cookies**. 7. Click **OK**.
Netscape Communicator or Navigator 4.5 or higher	1. Select **Edit**. 2. Select **Preferences**. 3. Click **Advanced**. 4. Click **Accept all cookies**. 5. Click **OK**.
Netscape Communicator or Navigator 6.1 or higher	1. Select **Edit**. 2. Select **Preferences**. 3. Select **Privacy & Security**. 4. Select **Cookies**. 5. Select **Enable All Cookies**.

Enable Java

Browser	Steps
Internet Explorer 5.0 or higher	1. Select **Tools**. 2. Select **Internet Options**. 3. Select the **Advanced** tab. 4. Locate **Microsoft VM**. 5. Make sure the **Java console enabled** and **Java logging enabled** boxes are checked. 6. Click **OK**. 7. Restart your computer if you checked the **Java console enabled** box.
Netscape Communicator or Navigator 4.5 or higher	1. Select **Edit** 2. Select **Preferences**. 3. Select **Advanced**. 4. Make sure the **Enable Java** and **Enable JavaScript** boxes are checked. 5. Click **OK**.

Set Cache to Always Reload a Page

Browser	Steps
Internet Explorer 5.0 or higher	1. Select **Tools**. 2. Select **Internet Options**. 3. Select the **General** tab. 4. Select **Settings** from within the **Temporary Internet Files** section. 5. Select the **Every visit to the page** button. 6. Click **OK**.
Netscape Communicator or Navigator 4.5 or higher	1. Select **Edit** 2. Select **Preferences**. 2. Click the + or → icon next to the **Advanced** to see more options. 3. Select **Cache**. 4. Select the **Every time** button at the bottom. 5. Click **OK**.

Plug-Ins

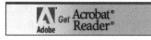 **Adobe Acrobat Reader**—With the free Acrobat Reader software you can view and print Adobe PDF files. Many Evolve products offer student and instructor manuals, checklists, and more in this format!

Download at: http://www.adobe.com

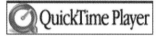 **Apple QuickTime**—Install this to hear word pronunciations, heart and lung sounds, and many other helpful audio clips within Evolve Online Courses!

Download at: http://www.apple.com

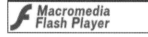 **Macromedia Flash Player**—This player will enhance your viewing of many Evolve web pages, as well as educational short-form to long-form animation within the Evolve Learning System!

Download at: http://www.macromedia.com

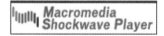 **Macromedia Shockwave Player**—Shockwave is best for viewing the many interactive learning activities within Evolve Online Courses!

Download at: http://www.macromedia.com

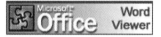 **Microsoft Word Viewer**—With this viewer Microsoft Word users can share documents with those who don't have Word, and users without Word can open and view Word documents. Many Evolve products have testbank, student and instructor manuals, and other documents available for downloading and viewing on your own computer!

Download at: http://www.microsoft.com

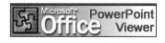 **Microsoft PowerPoint Viewer**—View PowerPoint 97, 2000, and 2002 presentations even if you don't have PowerPoint with this viewer. Many Evolve products have slides available for downloading and viewing on your own computer!

Download at: http://www.microsoft.com

Support Information

Live support is available to customers in the United States and Canada from 7:30 a.m. to 7:00 p.m. (Central Time), Monday through Friday by calling, **1-800-401-9962**. You can also send an email to evolve-support@elsevier.com.

There is also **24/7 support information** available on the Evolve website (http://evolve.elsevier.com), including:

- Guided Tours
- Tutorials
- Frequently Asked Questions (FAQs)
- Online Copies of Course User Guides
- And much more!

A QUICK TOUR

Welcome to *Virtual Clinical Excursions—Obstetrics-Pediatrics*, a virtual hospital setting in which you can work with multiple complex patient simulations and also learn to access and evaluate the information resources that are essential for high-quality patient care.

The virtual hospital, Pacific View Regional Hospital, has realistic architecture and access to patient rooms, a Nurses' Station, and a Medication Room.

■ BEFORE YOU START

Make sure you have your textbook nearby when you use the *Virtual Clinical Excursions—Obstetrics-Pediatrics* CD. You will want to consult topic areas in your textbook frequently while working with the CD and using this workbook.

■ HOW TO SIGN IN

- First, enter your name on the Student Nurse identification badge.
- Now select a period of care. The screen gives you four periods of care from which to choose. In Periods of Care 1 through 3, you can actively engage in patient assessment, entry of data in the electronic patient record (EPR), and medication administration. Period of Care 4 presents the day in review. Click on the appropriate period of care. (For this quick tour, choose **Period of Care 2**.)
- This takes you to the Patient List screen (see example on page 11). Note that the virtual time is provided in the box at the lower left corner of the screen (1115, since we chose Period of Care 2).

Note: If you choose to work during Period of Care 4: 1900-2000, the Patient List screen will not appear since you are not able to visit patients or administer medications during the shift. Instead, you are taken directly to the Nurses' Station, where the records of all the patients on the floor are available for your review.

■ **PATIENT LIST**

OBSTETRICS UNIT

Dorothy Grant (Room 201)
30-week intrauterine pregnancy—A young Caucasian multipara admitted with abdominal trauma following a domestic violence incident. Her complications include preterm labor and extensive social issues such as acquiring safe housing for her family upon discharge.

Stacey Crider (Room 202)
27-week intrauterine pregnancy—A young Native American primigravida admitted for intravenous tocolysis, bacterial vaginosis, and poorly controlled insulin-dependent gestational diabetes. Strained family relationships and social isolation complicate this patient's ability to comply with strict dietary requirements and prenatal care.

Kelly Brady (Room 203)
26-week intrauterine pregnancy—A 35-year-old Caucasian primigravida urgently admitted for progressive symptoms of preeclampsia. A history of inadequate coping with major life stressors leave her at risk for a recurrence of depression as she faces a diagnosis of HELLP syndrome and the delivery of a severely premature infant.

Maggie Gardner (Room 204)
22-week intrauterine pregnancy—A 41-year-old African-American multigravida admitted for a high-risk pregnancy evaluation and rule out diagnosis of systemic lupus erythematosus. Coping with chronic pain, fatigue, and a history of multiple miscarriages contribute to an anxiety disorder and the need for social service intervention.

Gabriela Valenzuela (Room 205)
34-week intrauterine pregnancy—A young Hispanic primigravida with a history of mitral valve prolapse admitted for uterine cramping and vaginal bleeding suggestive of placental abruption following an unrestrained motor vehicle accident. Her needs include staff support for an unprepared-for labor and possible preterm birth.

Laura Wilson (Room 206)
37-week intrauterine pregnancy—A teenage Caucasian primigravida urgently admitted after being found unconscious at home. Her complications include HIV-positive status and chronic polysubstance abuse. Unrealistic expectations of parenthood and living with a chronic illness combined with strained family relations prompt comprehensive social and psychiatric evaluations initiated on the day of simulation.

PEDIATRICS UNIT

George Gonzalez (Room 301)
Diabetic ketoacidosis—An 11-year-old Hispanic male admitted for stabilization of blood sugar and diabetic re-education associated with his diagnosis of type 1 diabetes mellitus. This patient's poor compliance with insulin therapy and dietary regime have resulted in frequent and repeated hospital admissions for DKA.

Tommy Douglas (Room 302)
Traumatic brain injury—A 6-year-old Caucasian male transferred from the Pediatric Intensive Care Unit in preparation for organ donation. This patient is status post ventriculostomy with negative intracerebral blood flow and requires extensive hemodynamic monitoring and support along with compassionate family care.

Carrie Richards (Room 303)
Bronchiolitis—A $3\frac{1}{2}$-month-old African-American female admitted with respiratory distress due to respiratory syncytial virus, along with dehydration and an inadequate nutritional status. Parent education and support are among her primary needs.

Stephanie Brown (Room 304)
Meningitis—A 3-year-old African-American female with a history of spastic cerebral palsy admitted for intravenous antibiotic therapy, neurological monitoring, and support for a diagnosis of acute meningitis. Maintenance of physical and occupational programs addressing her mobility limitations complicate her acute care stay.

Tiffany Sheldon (Room 305)
Anorexia nervosa—A 14-year-old Caucasian female admitted for dehydration, electrolyte imbalance, and malnutrition following a syncope episode at home. This patient has a history of eating disorders, which have resulted in multiple hospital admissions and strained family dynamics between mother and daughter.

Virtual Clinical Excursions 3.0 : Obstetric Patient Set

Patient List

	Patient Name	Room	MRN	Clinical Report
☑	Dorothy Grant	201	1868096	Get Report
☐	Stacey Crider	202	1868065	Get Report
☐	Kelly Brady	203	1868073	Get Report
☐	Maggie Gardner	204	1868085	Get Report
☐	Gabriela Valenzuela	205	1868090	Get Report
☐	Laura Wilson	206	1868098	Get Report

Please select all the patients you will be caring for this period of care. Once you have exited the patient list, you will not be able to change your current selections or select new patients to care for.

0730   Go to Nurses' Station

■ HOW TO SELECT A PATIENT

- You can choose one or more patients to work with from the Patient List by clicking the box to the left of the patient name(s). (In order to receive a scorecard for a patient, the patient must be selected before proceeding to the Nurses' Station.)
- Click on **Get Report** to the right of the medical records number (MRN) to view a summary of the patient's care during the 12-hour period before your arrival on the unit.
- After reviewing the report, click on **Return to Patient List**.
- When you are ready to begin your care, click on **Go to Nurses' Station** in the right lower corner.

■ HOW TO FIND A PATIENT'S RECORDS

NURSES' STATION

Within the Nurses' Station, you will see:

1. A clipboard that contains the patient list for that floor.
2. A chart rack with patient charts labeled by room number, a notebook labeled Kardex, and a notebook labeled MAR (Medication Administration Record).
3. A desktop computer with access to the Electronic Patient Record (EPR).
4. A tool bar across the top of the screen that can also be used to access the Patient List, EPR, Chart, MAR, and Kardex. This tool bar is also accessible from each patient's room.
5. A Drug Guide containing information about the medications you are able to administer to your patients.

As you run your cursor over an item, it will be highlighted. To select, simply double-click on the item. As you use these resources, you will always be able to return to the Nurses' Station by clicking on the **Return to Nurses' Station** bar located in the right lower corner of your screen.

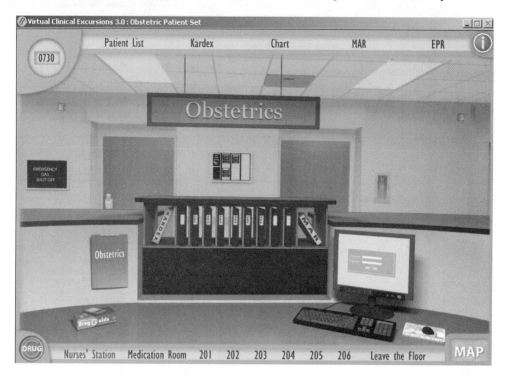

MEDICATION ADMINISTRATION RECORD (MAR)

The MAR icon located in the tool bar at the top of your screen accesses current 24-hour medications for each patient. Click on the icon and the MAR will open. (*Note:* You can also access the MAR by clicking on the blue MAR notebook on the far right side of the book rack in the center of the screen.) Within the MAR, tabs on the right side of the screen allow you to select patients by room number. Be careful to make sure you select the correct tab number for *your* patient rather than simply reading the first record that appears after the MAR opens. Each MAR sheet lists the following:

- Medications
- Route and dosage of medications
- Times of administration of medication

		Virtual Clinical Excursions 3.0 : Obstetric Patient Set			

Pacific View Regional Hospital

6475 E. Duke Avenue

MRN: 1868096   **Room:** 201
Patient: Dorothy Grant
Sex: Female   **Age:** 25
Physician: John Shelby, M.D.

Medication Administration Record
Wednesday

START	STOP	MEDICATION	0701-1900	1901-0700
Wed 0345		Lactated Ringer's 1000 mL IV continuous	1400	
Wed 0730	Wed 1930	Betamethasone 12 mg IM every 12 hours for 2 doses, dose #1	0730	1930
Wed 0730		Prenatal multivitamin 1 PO daily	0800	

0730   Return to Nurses' Station

201   202   203   204   205   206

Note: The MAR changes each day. Expired MARs are stored in the patients' charts.

CHARTS

To access patient charts, either click on the **Chart** icon at the top of your screen or anywhere within the chart rack in the center of the Nurses' Station screen. When the close-up view appears, the individual charts are labeled by room number. To open a chart, click on the room number of the patient whose chart you wish to review. The patient's name and allergies will appear, along with a list of tabs on the right side of the screen, allowing you to view the following data:

- Allergies
- Physician's Orders
- Physician's Notes
- Nurse's Notes
- Laboratory Reports
- Diagnostic Reports
- Surgical Reports
- Consultations

- Patient Education
- History and Physical
- Nursing Admission
- Expired MARs
- Consents
- Mental Health
- Admissions
- Emergency Department

Information appears in real time. The entries are in reverse chronological order, so use the down arrow at the right side of the chart page to scroll down to view previous entries. Flip from tab to tab to view multiple data fields or click on the **Return to Nurses' Station** bar in the lower right corner of the screen to exit the chart.

Virtual Clinical Excursions 3.0 : Obstetric Patient Set

Pacific View Regional Hospital

6475 E. Duke Avenue

MRN: 1868096	Room: 201
Patient: Dorothy Grant	
Sex: Female	Age: 25
Physician: John Shelby, M.D.	

Physician's Progress Notes

Day/Time	Notes	Signature
Wed 0730	25-year-old Caucasian female, G5, P3, AB 1, 30 weeks gestation, seen in ED for blunt abdominal trauma secondary to husband hitting and kicking abdomen of patient. Fundal height 29 cm. Ecchymosis and abrasions apparent on left lower abdomen and forearms. Remainder of physical examination WNL. OB ultrasound revealed normal fundal placement of placenta with no evidence of abruption. Fetus active with FHR in 130s. Admitted for observation. Mild contractions started approximately 2 hours after admission. Plan: 1. IV LR 500 mL bolus, then at 125 mL/hr. 2. Tocolysis if contractions continue. 3. Social services and Psychiatric consult. 4. Rho(D)Immune globulin for O negative blood type (patient missed her 28 week appointment and did not receive the Rho(D)Immune globulin at that time). 5. Betamethasone now and again in 12 hours if not delivered.	*Albert Song, M.D.*

Tabs: Allergies, Physician's Orders, Physician's Notes, Nurse's Notes, Laboratory Reports, Diagnostic Reports, Surgical Reports, Consultations, Patient Education, History and Physical, Nursing Admission, Expired MARs, Consents, Mental Health, Admissions, Emergency Department

0731

Return to Nurses' Station

ELECTRONIC PATIENT RECORD (EPR)

The EPR can be accessed from the computer in the Nurses' Station or from the EPR icon located in the tool bar at the top of your screen. To access a patient's EPR:
- Click on either the computer screen or the **EPR** icon.
- Your user name and password are automatically filled in.
- Click on **Login** to enter the EPR.

The EPR used in Pacific View Regional Hospital represents a composite of commercial versions being used in hospitals. You can access the EPR:
- for a patient (by room number).
- to review existing data.
- to enter data you collect while working with a patient.

The EPR is updated daily, so no matter what day or part of a shift you are working, there will be a current EPR with the patient's data from the past days of the current hospital stay. This type of simulated EPR allows you to examine how data for different attributes have changed over time, as well as to examine data for all of a patient's attributes at a particular time. The EPR is fully functional (as it is in a real-life hospital). You can enter such data as blood pressure, breath sounds, and certain treatments. The EPR will not, however, allow you to enter data for a previous time period. Use the arrows at the bottom of the screen to move forward and backward in time.

Virtual Clinical Excursions 3.0 : Obstetric Patient Set				
Patient: 201 Category: Vital Signs				**0731**
Name: Dorothy Grant	Wed 0345	Wed 0400	Wed 0500	Code Meanings
PAIN: LOCATION	A	A	A	A Abdomen
PAIN: RATING	1	1	2-3	Ar Arm
PAIN: CHARACTERISTICS	A	D	I	B Back
PAIN: VOCAL CUES		NN	NN	C Chest
PAIN: FACIAL CUES			FC2	Ft Foot
PAIN: BODILY CUES				H Head
PAIN: SYSTEM CUES	NN			Hd Hand
PAIN: FUNCTIONAL EFFECTS				L Left
PAIN: PREDISPOSING FACTORS		NN	NN	Lg Leg
PAIN: RELIEVING FACTORS		NN	NN	Lw Lower
PCA				N Neck
TEMPERATURE (F)		97.6		NN See Nurses notes
TEMPERATURE (C)				OS Operative site
MODE OF MEASUREMENT		O		Or See Physicians orders
SYSTOLIC PRESSURE		126		PN See Progress notes
DIASTOLIC PRESSURE		66		R Right
BP MODE OF MEASUREMENT		NIBP		Up Upper
HEART RATE		72		
RESPIRATORY RATE		18		
SpO2 (%)				
BLOOD GLUCOSE				
WEIGHT				
HEIGHT				

◄   ►   Exit EPR

At the top of the EPR screen, you can choose patients by their room numbers. In addition, you have access to 17 different categories of patient data. To change patients or data categories, click the down arrow to the right of the room number or category.

The categories of patient data in the EPR as as follows:

- Vital Signs
- Respiratory
- Cardiovascular
- Neurologic
- Gastrointestinal
- Excretory
- Musculoskeletal
- Integumentary
- Reproductive
- Psychosocial
- Wounds and Drains
- Activity
- Hygiene and Comfort
- Safety
- Nutrition
- IV
- Intake and Output

Remember, each hospital selects its own codes. The codes used in the EPR at Pacific View Regional Hospital may be different from ones you have seen in clinical rotations that have computerized patient records. Take some time to acquaint yourself with the codes. Within the Vital Signs category, click on any item in the left column (e.g., heart rate). In the far-right column, you will see a list of code meanings for the possible findings and/or descriptors for that assessment area.

You will use the codes to record the data you collect as you work with patients. Click on the box in the last time column to the right of the data and wait for the code meanings applicable to that entry to appear. Select the appropriate code to describe your assessment findings and type it in the box. (*Note:* If no cursor appears within the box, click on the box again until the blue shading disappears and the blinking cursor appears.) Once the data are typed in this box, they are entered into the patient's record for this period of care only.

To leave the EPR, click on **Exit EPR** in the bottom right corner of the screen.

■ **VISITING A PATIENT**

From the Nurses' Station, click on the room number of the patient you wish to visit in the tool bar at the bottom of your screen. Once you are inside the room, you will see a still photo of your patient in the top left corner. To verify that this is the patient you have chosen, click on the **Check Armband** icon to the right of the photo. The patient's identification data will appear. If you click on **Check Allergies** (the next icon to the right), a list of the patient's allergies (if any) will replace the photo.

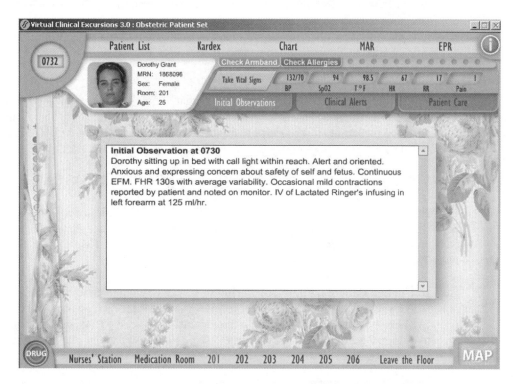

Also located in the patient's room are multiple icons you may use to assess the patient or the patient's medications. A clock is provided in the upper left corner of the room to monitor your progress in real time.

- The tool bar across the top of the screen allows you to check the **Patient List**, access the **EPR** to check or enter data, and view the patient's **Chart**, **MAR**, or **Kardex**.

- The **Take Vital Signs** icon allows you to measure the patient's up-to-the-minute blood pressure, oxygen saturation, temperature, heart rate, respiratory rate, and pain level.

- When you click on **Initial Observations**, a description appears in the text box under the patient's photo, allowing you a "look" at the patient as if you had just stepped in. To the right of this icon is **Clinical Alerts**, a resource that allows you to make decisions about priority medication interventions based on emerging data collected in real time. Check this screen throughout your period of care to avoid missing critical information related to recently ordered or STAT medications.

- Clicking on the **Patient Care** icon opens up three specific learning environments within the patient room: **Physical Assessment**, **Nurse-Client Interactions**, and **Medication Administration**.

- To perform a **Physical Assessment**, choose a body area (such as **Head & Neck**) by clicking on the appropriate icon in the column of yellow buttons. This activates a list of system subcategories for that body area (e.g., see **Sensory**, **Neurologic**, etc. in the green boxes). After you click on the system that you wish to evaluate, a still photo and text box appear, describing the assessment findings. The still photo is a "snapshot" of how an assessment of this area might be done or what the finding might look like. For every body area, there is also an **Equipment** button located on the far right of the screen.

- To the right of the Physical Assessment icon is **Nurse-Client Interactions**. Clicking on this icon will reveal the times and titles of any videos available for viewing. (*Note:* If the video you wish to see is not listed, this means you have not yet reached the correct virtual time to view that video. Check the virtual clock; you may return to access the video once its designated time has occurred—as long as you do so within the corresponding period of care.) To view a listed video, click on the white arrow to the right of the video title. Use the square control buttons below the video to start, stop, pause, rewind, or fast-forward the action or to mute the sound.

- **Medication Administration** is the pathway that allows you to review and administer medications to a patient after you have prepared them in the Medication Room. This process is addressed further in *How to Prepare Medications* (pages 19-20) and in *Medications* (pages 26-30).

■ HOW TO QUIT, CHANGE PATIENTS, OR CHANGE PERIOD OF CARE

How to Quit: From most screens, you may click the **Leave the Floor** icon on the bottom tool bar to the right of the patient room numbers. (*Note:* From some screens, you will first need to click an **Exit** button or **Return to Nurses' Station** before clicking **Leave the Floor**.) When the Floor Menu appears, click **Exit** to leave the program.

How to Change Patients, Floors, or Period of Care: To change patients, simply click on the new patient's room number. (You cannot receive a scorecard for a new patient, however, unless you have already selected that patient on the Patient List screen.) To change to a new period of care, to change floors, or to restart the virtual clock for a new patient, click the **Leave the Floor** icon and then **Restart**.

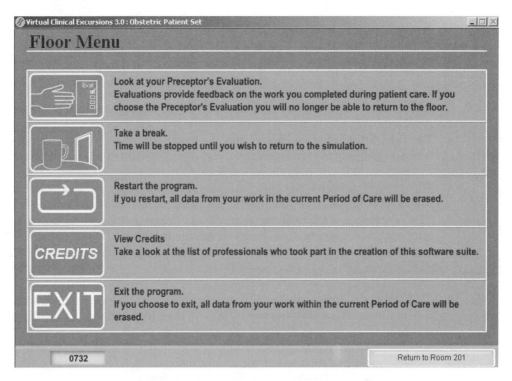

■ HOW TO PREPARE MEDICATIONS

From the Nurses' Station or the patient's room, you can access the Medication Room by clicking on the icon in the tool bar at the bottom of your screen to the left of the patient room numbers.

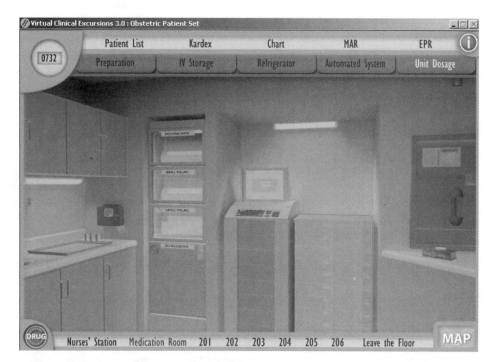

In the Medication Room you have access to the following (from left to right):

- A preparation area is located on the counter under the cabinets. To begin the medication preparation process, click on the tray on the counter or click on the **Preparation** icon at the top of the screen. The next screen leads you through a preparation sequence (called the Preparation Wizard) to prepare medications one at a time for administration to a patient. However, no medication has been selected at this time. We will do this while working with a patient in *A Detailed Tour*. To exit this screen, click on **View the Medication Room**.

- To the right of the cabinets (and above the refrigerator), IV storage bins are provided. Click on the bins themselves or on the **IV Storage** icon at the top of the screen. The bins are labeled **Microinfusion**, **Small Volume**, and **Large Volume**. Click on an individual bin to see a list of its contents. No medications are available in the bins at this time, but if they were, you could click on an individual medication and its label would appear to the right under the patient's name. Next, you would click **Put Medication on Tray**. If you ever change your mind or choose the incorrect medication, you can reverse your actions by clicking on **Put Medication in Bin**. Click **Close Bin** in the right bottom corner to exit. **View Medication Room** brings you back to a full view of the entire room.

- A refrigerator is located under the IV storage bins to hold any medications that must be stored below room temperature. Click on it to remove your medications; then click **Close Door**. You can also access this area by clicking the **Refrigerator** icon at the top of the screen.

- To prepare controlled substances, click the **Automated System** icon at the top of the screen or click the computer monitor located to the right of the IV storage bins. A login screen will appear; your name and password are automatically filled in. Click **Login**. Select a patient to log medications out for; then select the drawer you wish to open. Click **Open Drawer**, choose **Put Medication on Tray**, and then click **Close Drawer**.

- Next to the Automated System is a set of drawers identified by patient room number. To access these, click on the drawers themselves or on the **Unit Dosage** icon at the top of the screen. This provides a close-up view of the drawers. Click on the room number of the patient you are working with to open that drawer. Next, click on the medication you would like to prepare for the patient, and a label appears to the right under the patient's name, listing strength, units, and dosage per unit. You can **Open** and **Close** this medication label by clicking the appropriate icon. To exit, click **Close Drawer**; then click **View Medication Room**.

At any time, you can learn about a medication you wish to prepare for a patient by clicking on the **Drug** icon in the bottom left corner of the medication room screen or by clicking the **Drug Guide** book on the counter to the right of the unit dosage drawers. The **Drug Guide** provides information about the medications commonly included in nursing drug handbooks. Nutritional supplements and maintenance intravenous fluid preparations are not included.

To access the MAR to review the medications ordered for a patient, click on the **MAR** icon located in the tool bar at the top of your screen. You may also click the **Review MAR** icon in the tool bar at the bottom of your screen from inside each medication storage area.

After you have chosen and prepared your medications, return to the patient's room to administer them by clicking on the room number in the bottom tool bar. Once inside the patient's room, click on **Medication Administration** and follow the administration sequence.

■ PRECEPTOR'S EVALUATIONS

When you have finished a session, click on **Leave the Floor** to go to the Floor Menu. At this point, you can click on the icon next to **Look at your Preceptor's Evaluation** to receive a scorecard that provides feedback on the work you completed during patient care.

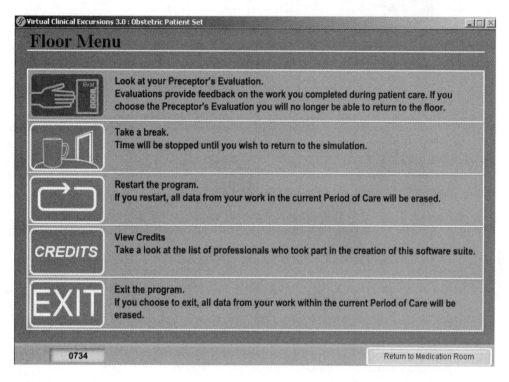

Evaluations are available for each patient you signed in for. Click on any of the **Medication Scorecard** icons to see an example. The scorecard compares the medications you administered to a patient during a period of care with what should have been administered. Table A lists the correct medications. Table B lists any medications that were administered incorrectly.

Not every medication listed on the MAR should be given. For example, a patient might have an allergy to a drug that was ordered, or a medication might have been improperly transcribed to the MAR. Predetermined medication "errors" embedded within the program challenge you to exercise critical thinking skills and professional judgment when deciding to administer a medication, just as you would in a real hospital. Use all your available resources, such as the patient's chart and the MAR, to make your decision.

Table C lists the resources that were available to assist you in medication administration, and it documents whether and when you accessed these resources. For example, did you check the patient armband or perform a check of vital signs? If so, when?

You can click **Print** to get a copy of this report if needed. Click **Return to Evaluations** when finished.

■ FLOOR MAP

To get a general sense of your location within the hospital, click on the **Map** icon found in the lower right corner of most of the screens in the *Virtual Clinical Excursions—Obstetrics-Pediatrics* program. A floor map will appear, showing the layout of the floor you are currently on, as well as a directory of the patients and services on that floor. As you move your cursor over the directory list, the location of each room is highlighted (and vice versa). The floor map can be accessed from the Nurses' Station, Medication Room, and each patient's room.

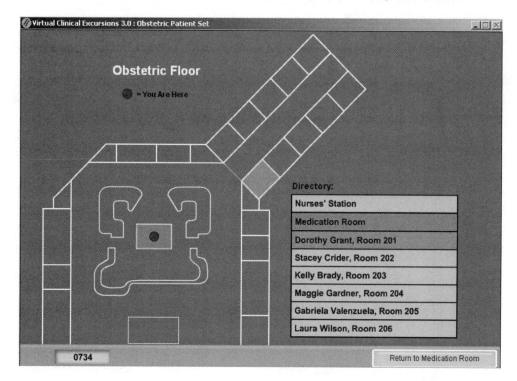

A DETAILED TOUR

If you wish to more thoroughly understand the capabilities of *Virtual Clinical Excursions—Obstetrics-Pediatrics*, take a detailed tour by completing the following section. During this tour, we will work with a specific patient to introduce you to all the different components and learning opportunities available within the software.

■ WORKING WITH A PATIENT

Sign in to work on the Obstetrics Floor for Period of Care 1 (0730-0815). From the Patient List, select Dorothy Grant in Room 201; however, do not go to the Nurses' Station yet.

	Patient Name	Room	MRN	Clinical Report
☑	Dorothy Grant	201	1868096	Get Report
☐	Stacey Crider	202	1868065	Get Report
☐	Kelly Brady	203	1868073	Get Report
☐	Maggie Gardner	204	1868085	Get Report
☐	Gabriela Valenzuela	205	1868090	Get Report
☐	Laura Wilson	206	1868098	Get Report

Patient List

Please select all the patients you will be caring for this period of care. Once you have exited the patient list, you will not be able to change your current selections or select new patients to care for.

0730   Go to Nurses' Station

■ REPORT

In hospitals, when one shift ends and another begins, the outgoing nurse who attended a patient will give a verbal and sometimes a written summary of that patient's condition to the incoming nurse who will assume care for the patient. This summary is called a report and is an important source of data to provide an overview of a patient. Your first task is to get clinical report on Dorothy Grant. To do this, click **Get Report** in the far right column in this patient's row. From this summary, identify the problems and areas of concern that you will need to address for this patient.

When you have finished reading the report and noting any areas of concern, click **Go to Nurses' Station**.

■ CHARTS

You can access Dorothy Grant's chart from the Nurses' Station or from the patient's room (201). We will access it from the Nurses' Station: Click on the chart rack or on the **Chart** icon in the tool bar at the top of your screen. Next, click on the chart labeled **201** to open the medical record for Dorothy Grant. Click on the **Emergency Department** tab to view a record of why this patient was admitted.

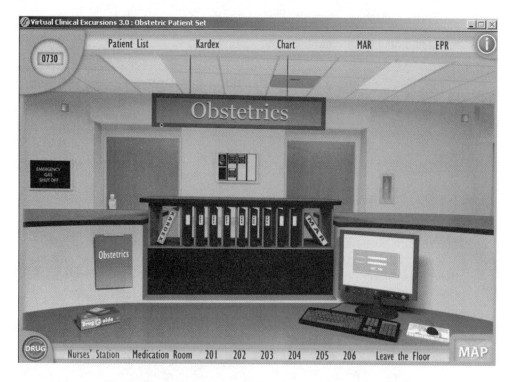

How many days has Dorothy Grant been in the hospital?

What tests were done upon her arrival in the Emergency Department and why?

What was the reason for her admission?

You should also click on **Surgical Reports** to learn whether any procedures were performed and when. Finally, review the **Nursing Admission** and **History and Physical** tabs to view information on the health history of this patient. When you are done reviewing the chart, click **Return to Nurses' Station**.

■ MEDICATIONS

Open the Medication Administration Record (MAR) by clicking on the **MAR** icon in the tool bar at the top of your screen. *Remember:* The MAR automatically opens to the first occupied room number on the floor. Since you need to access Dorothy Grant's MAR, click on tab **201** (her room number). Always make sure you are giving the *Right Drug to the Right Patient!*

Examine the list of medications prescribed for Dorothy Grant. Write down the medications that need to be given during this period of care (0730-0815). For each medication, note the dosage, route, and time in the chart below.

Time	Medication	Dosage	Route

Click on **Return to Nurses' Station**. Next, click on **201** on the bottom tool bar and then verify that you are indeed in Dorothy Grant's room. Select **Clinical Alerts** (the icon to the right of Initial Observations) to check for any emerging data that might affect your medication administration priorities. Go to the patient's chart (click on the **Chart** icon; then click on **201**). When the chart opens, select the **Physician's Orders** tab.

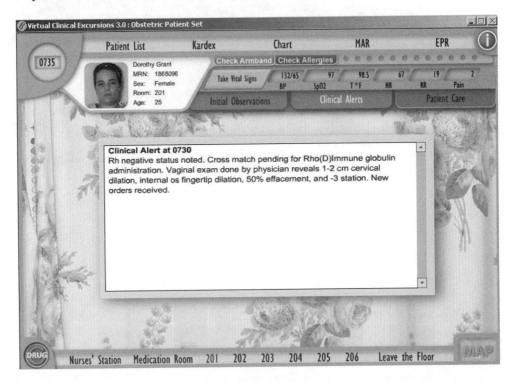

Review the orders. Have any new medications been ordered? Return to the MAR (click **Return to Room 201**; then click **MAR**). Verify that the new medications have been correctly transcribed to the MAR. Mistakes are sometimes made in the transcription process in the hospital setting, and it is sound practice to double-check any new order.

Are there any patient assessments you will need to perform before administering these medications? If so, return to Room 201 and complete those before proceeding.

Now click on the **Medication Room** icon in the tool bar at the bottom of your screen to locate and prepare the medications for Dorothy Grant.

In the Medication Room, you must access the medications for Dorothy Grant from the specific dispensing system in which each medication is stored. Locate each medication that needs to be given in this time period and click on **Put Medication on Tray** as appropriate. (*Hint:* Look in Unit Dosage drawer first.) When you are finished, click on **Close Drawer** and then on **View Medication Room**. Now click on the medication tray on the counter on the left side of the medication room screen to begin preparing the medications you have selected. (*Note:* Instead of clicking on the tray, you can click **Preparation** at top of screen.)

In the preparation area, you should see a list of the medications you put on the tray in the previous steps. Click on the first medication and then click **Prepare**. Follow the onscreen instructions of the Preparation Wizard, providing any data requested. As an example, let's follow the preparation process for betamethasone, one of the medications due to be administered to Dorothy Grant during this period of care. To begin, click on **Betamethasone**; then click **Prepare**. Now work through the Preparation Wizard sequence as detailed below:

Amount of medication in the ampule: 5 mL
Enter the amount of medication you will draw up into a syringe: **3** mL
Click **Next**.
Select the patient you wish to set aside the medication for:
Click **Room 201, Dorothy Grant**.
Click **Finish**.
Click **Return to Medication Room**.

Follow this same basic process for the other medications due to be administered to Dorothy Grant during this period of care. (*Hint:* Look in **IV Storage** and **Automated System**.)

PREPARATION WIZARD EXCEPTIONS

- Some medications in *Virtual Clinical Excursions—Obstetrics-Pediatrics* are prepared by the pharmacy (e.g., IV antibiotics) and taken to the patient room as a whole. This is common practice in most hospitals.
- Blood products are not administered by students through the *Virtual Clinical Excursions—Obstetrics-Pediatrics* simulations since blood administration follows specific protocols not covered in this program.
- The *Virtual Clinical Excursions—Obstetrics-Pediatrics* simulations do not allow for mixing more than one type of medication, such as regular and Lente insulins, in the same syringe. In the clinical setting, when multiple types of insulin are ordered for a patient, the regular insulin is drawn up first, followed by the longer-acting insulin. Insulin is always administered in a special unit-marked syringe.

Now return to Room 201 (click on **201** on bottom tool bar) to administer Dorothy Grant's medications.

At any time during the medication administration process, you can perform a further review of systems, take vital signs, check information contained within the chart, or verify patient identity and allergies. Inside Dorothy Grant's room, click **Take Vital Signs**. (*Note:* These findings change over time to reflect the temporal changes you would find in a patient similar to Dorothy Grant.)

When you have gathered all the data you need, click on **Patient Care** and then select **Medication Administration**. After reviewing your medications, continue the administration process with the betamethasone ordered for Dorothy Grant. In the list of medications set aside for this patient, click to highlight **Betamethasone**. Next, click on the down arrow to the right of **Select** and choose **Administer** from the drop-down menu. This will activate the Administration Wizard. Complete the Wizard sequence as follows:

- Route: **Injection**
- Method: **Intramuscular**
- Site: **Any**
- Click **Administer to Patient** arrow.
- Would you like to document this administration in the MAR? **Yes**
- Click **Finish** arrow.

Selections are recorded by a tracking system and evaluated on a Medication Scorecard stored under Preceptor's Evaluations. This scorecard can be viewed, printed, and given to your instructor. To access the Preceptor's Evaluations, click on **Leave the Floor**. When the Floor Menu appears, click on the icon next to **Look at Your Preceptor's Evaluation**. From the list of evaluations, click on **Medication Scorecard** inside the box with Dorothy Grant's name.

■ MEDICATION SCORECARD

- First, review Table A. Was betamethasone given correctly? Did you give the other medications as ordered?
- Table B shows you which (if any) medications you gave incorrectly.
- Table C addresses the resources used for Dorothy Grant. Did you access the patient's chart, MAR, EPR, or Kardex as needed to make safe medication administration decisions?
- Did you check the patient's armband to verify her identity? Did you check whether your patient had any known allergies to medications? Were vital signs taken?

■ VITAL SIGNS

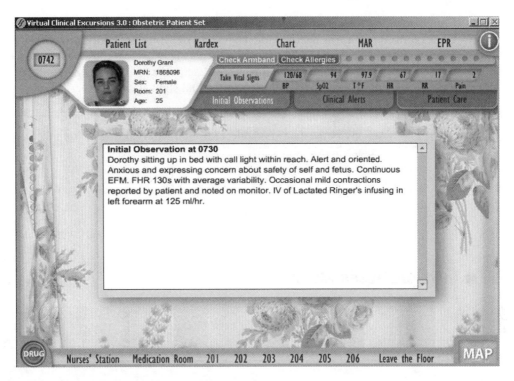

Vital signs, often considered the traditional signs of life, include body temperature, heart rate, respiratory rate, blood pressure, oxygen saturation of the blood, and the patient's experience of pain.

Inside Dorothy Grant's room, click **Take Vital Signs**. (*Remember:* You can take vital signs at any time. The data change over time to reflect the temporal changes you would find in a patient similar to Dorothy Grant.) Collect vital signs for this patient and record them in the following table. Note the time at which you collected each of these data.

Vital Signs	Findings/Time
Blood pressure	
O$_2$ saturation	
Heart rate	
Respiratory rate	
Temperature	
Pain rating	

After you are done, click on the **EPR** icon located in the tool bar at the top of the screen.

Complete the EPR Login screen as directed in *A Quick Tour* (see page 15 of this workbook). Click on the down arrow next to Patient and choose Dorothy Grant's room number **201**. Select **Vital Signs** as the category. Next, record the vital signs data you just collected in the last column. (*Note:* If you need help with this process, see page 16.) Now compare these findings with the data you collected earlier for this patient's vital signs. Use these earlier findings to establish a baseline for each of the vital signs.

      a. Are any of the data you collected significantly different from the baseline for a particular vital sign?

          Circle One: Yes   No

      b. If "Yes," which data are different?

■ PHYSICAL ASSESSMENT

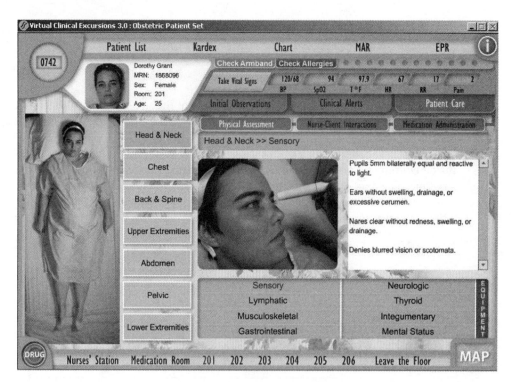

After you have finished examining the EPR for vital signs, click **Exit EPR** to return to Room 201. Click **Patient Care** and then **Physical Assessment**. Think about what information you received in report, as well as what you may have learned about this patient from the chart. What area(s) of examination should you pay most attention to at this time? Is there any equipment you should be monitoring? Conduct a physical assessment of the body areas and systems that you consider priorities for Dorothy Grant. For example, select **Head & Neck**; then click on and assess **Mental Status** and **Equipment**. Complete any other assessment(s) you think are necessary at this time. In the following table, record the data you collected during this examination.

Area of Examination	Findings
Head & Neck Mental Status	
Head & Neck Equipment	

After you have finished collecting these data, return to the EPR. Compare the data that were already in the record with those you just collected.

    a.   Are any of the data you collected significantly different from the baselines for this patient?

        Circle One: Yes   No

    b.   If "Yes," which data are different?

■ NURSE-CLIENT INTERACTIONS

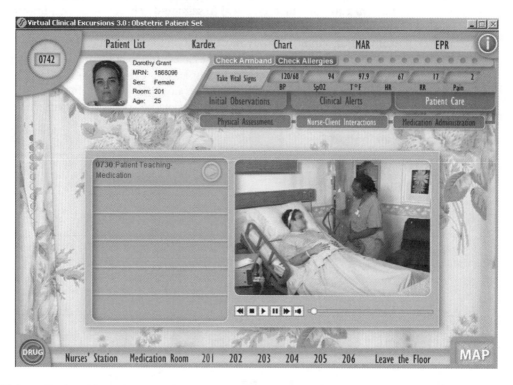

Click on **Patient Care** from inside Dorothy Grant's room (201). Now click on **Nurse-Client Interactions** to access a short video titled **Patient Teaching—Medication**, which is available for viewing at 0730 (based on the virtual clock in the upper left corner of your screen). To begin the video, click on the arrow next to its title. You will observe a nurse communicating with Dorothy Grant. There are many variations of nursing practice, some exemplifying "best" practice and some not. Note whether the nurse in this interaction displays professional behavior and compassionate care. Are her words congruent with what is going on with the patient? Does this interaction "feel right" to you? If not, how would you handle this situation differently? Explain.

Note: If the video you wish to view is not listed, this means you have not yet reached the correct virtual time to view that video. Check the virtual clock; you may return to access the video once its designated time has occurred—as long as you do so within the corresponding period of care.

At least one Nurse-Client Interactions video is available during each period of care. Viewing these videos can help you learn more about what is occurring with a patient at a certain time and also prompt you to discriminate between nurse communications that are ideal and those that need improvement. Compassionate care and the ability to communicate clearly are essential components of delivering quality nursing care, and it is during your clinical time that you will begin to refine these skills.

■ **COLLECTING AND EVALUATING DATA**

Each of the activities you perform in the Patient Care environment generates a great deal of assessment data. Remember that after you collect data, you can record your findings in the EPR. You can also review the EPR, patient's chart, videos, and MAR at any time. You will get plenty of practice collecting and then evaluating data in context of the patient's course.

Now, here's an important question for you:

> Did the previous sequence of exercises provide the most efficient way to assess Dorothy Grant?

For example, you went to the patient's room to get vital signs, then back to the EPR to enter data and compare your findings with extant data. Next, you went back to the patient's room to do a physical examination, then again back to the EPR to enter and review data. If this back-and-forth process of data collection and recording seemed inefficient, remember the following:

- Plan all of your nursing activities to maximize efficiency while at the same time optimizing quality of patient care. (Think about what data you might need to perform certain tasks. For example, do you need to check a heart rate before administering a cardiac medication or check an IV site before starting an infusion?)

- You collect a tremendous amount of data when you work with a patient. Very few people can accurately remember all these data for more than a few minutes. Develop efficient assessment skills, and record data as soon as possible after collecting them.

- Assessment data are only the starting point for the nursing process.

Make a clear distinction between these first exercises and how you actually provide nursing care. These initial exercises were designed to involve you actively in the use of different software components. This workbook focuses on sensible practices for implementing the nursing process in ways that ensure the highest quality care of patients.

Most important, remember that a human being changes through time, and that these changes include both the physical and psychosocial facets of a person as a living organism. Think about this for a moment. Some patients may change physically in a very short time (a patient with emerging myocardial infarction) or more slowly (a patient with a chronic illness). Patients' overall physical and psychosocial conditions may improve or deteriorate. They may have effective coping skills and familial support, or they may feel alone and full of despair. In fact, each individual is a complex mix of physical and psychosocial elements, and at least some of these elements usually change through time.

Thus it is crucial *not* to think of the nursing process as a simple one-time, five-step procedure:

- Assessment
- Nursing Diagnosis
- Planning
- Implementation
- Evaluation

Rather, the nursing process should be utilized as a creative and systematic approach to delivering nursing care. Furthermore, because all living organisms are constantly changing, we must apply the nursing process over and over. Each time we follow the nursing process for an individual patient, we refine our understanding of that patient's physical and psychosocial conditions based on collection and analysis of many different types of data. *Virtual Clinical Excursions—Obstetrics-Pediatrics* will help you develop both the creativity and the systematic approach needed to become a nurse who is equipped to deliver the highest quality care to all patients.

REDUCING MEDICATION ERRORS

Earlier in this detailed tour, you learned the basic steps of medication preparation and administration. The following simulations will allow you to practice those skills further—with an increased emphasis on reducing medication errors by using the Medication Scorecard to evaluate your work.

Sign in to work at Pacific View Regional Hospital for Period of Care 1. (*Note:* If you are already working with another patient or during another period of care, click on **Leave the Floor** and then **Restart the Program**; then sign in.)

From the Patient List, select Dorothy Grant. Then click on **Go to Nurses' Station**. Complete the following steps to prepare and administer medications to Dorothy Grant.

- Click on **Medication Room**.
- Click on **MAR** to determine prn medications that have been ordered for Dorothy Grant. (*Note:* You may click on **Review MAR** at any time to verify correct medication order. Remember to look at the patient name on the MAR to make sure you have the correct patient's record—you must click on the correct room number within the MAR.) Click on **Return to Medication Room** after reviewing the correct MAR.
- Click on **Unit Dosage** (or on the Unit Dosage cabinet); from the close-up view, click on drawer **201**.
- Select the medications you would like to administer. After each selection, click **Put Medication on Tray**. When you are finished selecting medications, click **Close Drawer**.
- Click **View Medication Room**.
- Click **Automated System** (or on the Automated System unit itself). Click **Login**.
- On the next screen, specify the correct patient and drawer location.
- Select the medication you would like to administer and click **Put Medication on Tray**. Repeat this process if you wish to administer other medications from the Automated System.
- When you are finished, click **Close Drawer**. At the bottom right corner of the next screen, click **View Medication Room**.
- From the Medication Room, click **Preparation** (or on the preparation tray).
- From the list of medications on your tray, choose the correct medication to administer.
- Click **Next**, specify the correct patient to administer this medication to, and click **Finish**.
- Repeat the previous two steps until all medications that you want to administer are prepared.
- You can click on **Review Your Medications** and then on **Return to Medication Room** when ready. Once you are back in the Medication Room, go directly to Dorothy Grant's room by clicking on **201** at the bottom of the screen.
- Inside the patient's room, administer the medication, utilizing the five rights of medication administration. After you have collected the appropriate assessment data and are ready for administration, click **Patient Care** and then **Medication Administration**. Verify that the correct patient and medication(s) appear in the left-hand window. Then click the down arrow next to Select. From the drop-down menu, select **Administer** and complete the Administration Wizard by providing any information requested. When the Wizard stops asking for information, click **Administer to Patient**. Specify **Yes** when asked whether this administration should be recorded in the MAR. Finally, click **Finish**.

■ **SELF-EVALUATION**

Now let's see how you did during your earlier medication administration!

- Click on **Leave the Floor** at the bottom of your screen. From the Floor Menu, select **Look at Your Preceptor's Evaluation**. Then click **Medication Scorecard**.

These resources will help you find out more about each patient's medications and possible sources of medication errors.

1. Start by examining Table A. These are the medications you should have given to Dorothy Grant during this period of care. If each of the medications in Table A has a ✓ by it, then you made no errors. Congratulations!

If there are some medications that have an X by them, then you made one or more medication errors.

Compare Tables A and B to determine which of the following types of errors you made: Wrong Dose, Wrong Route/Method/Site, or Wrong Time. Follow these steps:
   a. Find medications in Table A that were given incorrectly.
   b. Now see if those same medications are in Table B, which shows what you actually administered to Dorothy Grant.
   c. Comparing Tables A and B, match the Strength, Dose, Route/Method/Site, and Time for each medication you administered incorrectly.
   d. Then, using the form below, list the medications given incorrectly and mark the errors you made for each medication.

Medication	Strength	Dosage	Route	Method	Site	Time
	❏	❏	❏	❏	❏	❏
	❏	❏	❏	❏	❏	❏
	❏	❏	❏	❏	❏	❏
	❏	❏	❏	❏	❏	❏

2. To help you reduce future medication errors, consider the following list of possible reasons for errors.

   - Did not check drug against MAR for correct patient, correct date, correct time, correct drug, and correct dose.
   - Did not check drug dose against MAR three times.
   - Did not open the unit dose package in the patient's room.
   - Did not correctly identify the patient using two identifiers.
   - Did not administer the drug on time.
   - Did not verify patient allergies.
   - Did not check the patient's current condition or vital sign parameters.
   - Did not consider why the patient would be receiving this drug.
   - Did not question why the drug was in the patient's drawer.
   - Did not check the physician's order and/or check with the pharmacist when there was a question about the drug or dose.
   - Did not verify that no adverse effects had occurred from a previous dose.

Based on these possibilities, determine how you made each error and record the reason into the form below:

Medication	Reason for Error

3. Look again at Table B. Are there medications listed that are not in Table A? If so, you gave a medication to Dorothy Grant that she should not have received. Complete the following exercises to help you understand how such an error might have been made.

   a. Perhaps you gave a medication that was on Dorothy Grant's MAR for this period of care, without recognizing that a change had occurred in the patient's condition that should have caused you to reconsider. Review patient records as necessary and complete the following form:

Medication	Possible Reasons Not to Give This Medication

   b. Another possibility is that you gave Dorothy Grant a medication that should have been given at a different time. Check her MAR and complete the form below to determine whether you made a Wrong Time error:

Medication	Given to Dorothy Grant at What Time	Should Have Been Given at What Time

c. Maybe you gave another patient's medication to Dorothy Grant. In this case, you made a Wrong Patient error. Check the MARs of other patients and use the form below to determine whether you made this type of error:

Medication	Given to Dorothy Grant	Should Have Been Given to

4. The Medication Scorecard provides some other interesting sources of information. For example, if there is a medication selected for Dorothy Grant but it was not given to her, there will be an X by that medication in Table A, but it will not appear in Table B. In that case, you might have given this medication to some other patient, which is another type of Wrong Patient error. To investigate further, look at Table D, which lists the medications you gave to other patients. See whether you can find any medications for Dorothy Grant that were given to another patient by mistake. Before making any decisions, be sure to cross-check the other patients' MAR because they may have had the same medication ordered. Use the following form to record your findings:

Medication	Should Have Been Given to Dorothy Grant	Given by Mistake to

5. Now take some time to review the exercises you just completed. Use the form below to create an overall analysis of what you have learned. Once again, record each of the medication errors you made, including the type of each error. Then, for each error you made, indicate specifically what you would do differently to prevent this type of error from occurring again.

Medication	Type of Error	Error Prevention Tactic

Submit this form to your instructor if required as a graded assignment, or simply use these exercises to improve your understanding of medication errors and how to reduce them.

Name: _____   Date: _____

The following icons are used throughout the workbook to help you quickly identify particular activities and assignments:

 Indicates a reading assignment—tells you which textbook chapter(s) you should read before starting each lesson

 Indicates a writing activity

 Marks the beginning of an interactive CD-ROM activity—signals you to open or return to your *Virtual Clinical Excursions—Obstetrics-Pediatrics* CD-ROM

 Indicates additional CD-ROM instructions

 Indicates questions and activities that require you to consult your textbook

 Indicates the approximate time required to complete an exercise

LESSON **1**

The Childbearing and Child-Rearing Family

/O⌒O Reading Assignment: The Childbearing and Child-Rearing Family (Chapter 3)

Patients: Dorothy Grant, Room 201
Stacey Crider, Room 202
Kelly Brady, Room 203
Maggie Gardner, Room 204
Gabriela Valenzuela, Room 205
Laura Wilson, Room 206

Goal: Demonstrate an understanding of how the family, community, and culture affects the pregnant woman.

Objectives:

* Assess and plan care for a patient from a specific culture.
* Explore how your background influences the care that you give to patients who have differing experiences in regard to community, family, or culture.
* Discuss the various types of families, communities, and cultures represented by each of the patients.

Exercise 1

CD-ROM Activity

15 minutes

Review pages 40-42 in your textbook and complete the following exercise regarding family types.

Read question 1 before starting this period of care. Fill in the table as you review each patient's chart.

- Sign in to work at Pacific View Regional Hospital on the Obstetrics Floor for Period of Care 1. (*Note*: If you are already in the virtual hospital from a previous exercise, click on **Leave the Floor** and then **Restart the Program** to get to the sign-in window.)
- From the Patient List, select all the patients to review.
- Click on **Go to Nurses' Station** and then on **Chart**.
- Click on Dorothy Grant's chart (**201**) to begin.
- Click on the **Admissions** tab and find the patient's marital status.
- Click on the **History and Physical** tab and review the Family History section.
- Once you have completed the column for Dorothy Grant in the table below, click on **Return to Nurses' Station** and review Stacey Crider's chart (**202**). Repeat this sequence until you have completed question 1.

1. Under each patient's name below, place an X to indicate that patient's type of family.

	Dorothy Grant	Stacey Crider	Kelly Brady	Maggie Gardner	Gabriela Valenzuela	Laura Wilson
Nuclear						
Single-income						
Multi-generational						
Blended						
High-risk						

2. Using what you learned in your chart review, combined with the information in your textbook, describe the type of family that Gabriela Valenzuela has.

3. Based on the information provided in your textbook, what type of family do you have? Describe how your family fits the description of the family type you have chosen.

 Review pages 44-46 in your textbook regarding various cultural and religious groups. Answer questions 4 through 9 regarding that material.

4. Among the Asian American culture, what is one form of medicine that is widely accepted? Give an example.

5. What do Native Americans believe in regard to health?

6. What is one barrier in providing health care to patients from the Middle Eastern culture?

7. In the Hispanic culture, _____ and _____ have a very strong association.

8. Based on your review of the information in the textbook, will you change your care for patients of differing cultures? If so, how? What community resources are available for patients of various cultures where you live?

Exercise 2

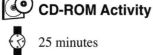 **CD-ROM Activity**

25 minutes

Culturally competent care is very important. As we review the various ways of providing culturally competent care, we will review two patients on the VCE.

- Sign in to work at Pacific View Regional Hospital on the Obstetrics Floor for Period of Care 1. (*Note*: If you are already in the virtual hospital from a previous exercise, click on **Leave the Floor** and then **Restart the Program** to get to the sign-in window.)
- From the Patient List, select Stacey Crider and Maggie Gardner.
- Click on **Go to Nurses' Station**.
- Click on **Chart** and then on **202**.
- Click on the **Nursing Admission** tab.
- Review Stacey Crider's Nursing Admission. (*Hint*: See the Role Relationships section.)

1. Identify a nursing diagnosis that would be appropriate for Stacey Crider and her family.

Maggie Gardner and her husband are very religious. According to the textbook, most members of the African-American culture have strong feelings about family, community, and religion. With this information in mind, complete the following activity and questions.

- Click on **Return to Nurses' Station**.
- Click on Room **204** at the bottom of the screen.
- Click on **Patient Care**.
- Click on **Nurse-Client Interactions**.
- Select and view the video titled **0730: Communicating Empathy**. (*Note*: If this video is not available, check the virtual clock to see whether enough time has elapsed. The video cannot be viewed before its specified time.)

2. What does Maggie Gardner's husband verbalize during this interaction that would correlate with the African-American population's deep sense of religion?

3. Based on your interactions with patients in the hospital where you have worked, describe your experience(s) with caring for someone of a different culture. What are some of the ideals that are different from your own? What barriers have you experienced to your care?

4. How comfortable are you with caring for patients from a different culture? Do you find yourself feeling judgmental or attempting to change others? What can you do to learn more about other cultures?

To further explore Jim and Maggie Gardner's spiritual perspective, return to the patient's chart.

- Click on **Chart** and then on **204**.
- Click on the **Consultations** tab.
- Review the Pastoral Care Spiritual Assessment and the Pastoral Consultation. (*Hint:* Be sure to scroll down to read all the pages in this section.)

5. What does Maggie Gardner "blame" her miscarriages on?

6. Based on your review, what is Maggie Gardner's perception of God?

7. Based on your review of Maggie Gardner's chart during this exercise, what is one underlying theme that you see in the Consultations, Nursing Admission, and History and Physical in regard to religion and this patient's perception of her situation?

LESSON **2**

Management of Fertility and Infertility

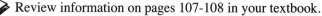

 Reading Assignment: Management of Fertility and Infertility (Chapter 10)

Patients: Stacey Crider, Room 202
Kelly Brady, Room 203
Maggie Gardner, Room 204
Gabriela Valenzuela, Room 205
Laura Wilson, Room 206

Goal: Demonstrate an understanding of reproductive system concerns, contraception options, and infertility.

Objectives:

- Identify reproductive concerns that can occur.
- Differentiate among the varying types of contraception available.
- Identify various methods of testing and treatment options that can be used for couples experiencing infertility concerns.

Exercise 1

CD-ROM Activity

10 minutes

Review information on pages 107-108 in your textbook.

1. What is a normal length for a menstrual cycle?

2. What are the criteria required to diagnose an individual with amenorrhea?

→ • Sign in to work at Pacific View Regional Hospital on the Obstetrics Floor for Period of Care 1. (*Note*: If you are already in the virtual hospital from a previous exercise, click on **Leave the Floor** and then **Restart the Program** to get to the sign-in window.)

• From the Patient List, select Stacey Crider.

• Click on **Go to Nurses' Station**.

• Click on **Chart** and then on **202**.

• Click on **History and Physical**.

• Review the patient's gynecologic history. (*Hint:* See the bottom of page 1.)

 3. Does Stacey Crider meet the textbook criteria for amenorrhea?

4. What is her history?

5. List three things that can cause amenorrhea.

Exercise 2

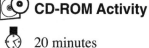 **CD-ROM Activity**

 20 minutes

Review pages 184-200 in the textbook.

1. What is contraception?

2. What is the primary consideration when recommending/evaluating methods of contraception?

→ • Sign in to work at Pacific View Regional Hospital on the Obstetrics Floor for Period of Care 1. (*Note*: If you are already in the virtual hospital from a previous exercise, click on **Leave the Floor** and then **Restart the Program** to get to the sign-in window.)

• From the Patient List, select Kelly Brady, Gabriela Valenzuela, and Laura Wilson.

• Click on **Go to Nurses' Station**.

• Click on **Chart** and then on **203** for Kelly Brady's chart.

• Review the **History and Physical**.

• Repeat the previous three steps for Gabriela Valenzuela and Laura Wilson.

3. Identify the birth control method each woman was using prior to her current pregnancy.

Kelly Brady

Gabriela Valenzuela

Laura Wilson

4. No contraceptive is _____ effective in preventing

_____.

5. Gabriela Valenzuela is Catholic. Which method would be appropriate for the nurse to discuss with her?

6. What does this method rely on?

7. Kelly Brady wants to use oral contraceptives while breastfeeding to prevent pregnancy. Which type of oral contraception is appropriate for her to use? Why?

8. Laura Wilson is HIV-positive. What is the most appropriate form of birth control for her? Why?

Exercise 3

CD-ROM Activity

20 minutes

Review pages 200-213 in your textbook.

1. _____ of the population of reproductive age has a problem with infertility.

2. In the _____ a natural decline in fertility begins.

3. List four factors that affect male fertility.

4. List three factors that affect female fertility.

➔ • Sign in to work at Pacific View Regional Hospital on the Obstetrics Floor for Period of Care 1. (*Note*: If you are already in the virtual hospital from a previous exercise, click on **Leave the Floor** and then **Restart the Program** to get to the sign-in window.)
   • From the Patient List, select Maggie Gardner.
   • Click on **Go to Nurses' Station**.
   • Click on **Chart** and then on **204**.
   • Review the **History and Physical**.

5. Maggie Gardner was married _____ years prior to conceiving the first time.

6. Based on the textbook reading, with which of the following would Maggie Gardner have been diagnosed if she had chosen to get treatment after a year of attempting to get pregnant?
   a. Primary infertility
   b. Secondary infertility

Review pages 204-209 in your textbook to answer the following questions.

7. What three tests can be completed on a male patient to determine the causes of infertility?

8. What four tests can be completed on a female patient to determine the causes of infertility?

9. What test is used to assess a couple to determine adequacy of coital technique?

10. What methods are available to assist an infertile couple to conceive?

11. What methods did Maggie Gardner and her husband use to assist in getting pregnant? (*Hint*: Review the OB history in the History and Physical.)

LESSON 3

Nutrition for Childbearing/ Prenatal Diagnostic Tests

Reading Assignment: Nutrition for Childbearing (Chapter 15)
Prenatal Diagnostic Tests (Chapter 16)
The Pregnant Woman with Complications (Chapter 26)

Patients: Kelly Brady, Room 203
Maggie Gardner, Room 204
Laura Wilson, Room 206

Goal: Demonstrate an understanding of the assessment of risk factors in pregnancy, including maternal and fetal nutritional aspects.

Objectives:

- Identify appropriate interventions for maintaining adequate maternal and fetal nutrition.
- Differentiate among the varying types of assessment techniques that can be used with both low- and high-risk pregnancy patients.
- Identify various methods of testing that can be used in high-risk pregnancies.

Exercise 1

CD-ROM Activity

 15 minutes

- Sign in to work at Pacific View Regional Hospital on the Obstetrics Floor for Period of Care 1. (*Note*: If you are already in the virtual hospital from a previous exercise, click on **Leave the Floor** and then **Restart the Program** to get to the sign-in window.)
- From the Patient List, select Maggie Gardner
- Click on **Go to Nurses' Station**.
- Click on **Chart** and then on **204**.
- Click on **Laboratory Reports**.

Review information regarding anemia on pages 212-214 and 657-658 in the textbook.

1. What were Maggie Gardner's hemoglobin and hematocrit levels on admission?

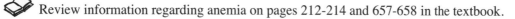

→ • Click on **History and Physical**.

2. What puts Maggie Gardner at a greater risk for developing anemia than the average pregnancy patient? (*Hint*: Review the Genetic Screening section of her History and Physical.)

3. What complication do women with anemia experience at a higher rate than those without anemia?

4. What is a normal hematocrit level for women who are pregnant?

5. What assessments, specifically related to an anemia diagnosis, need to be performed by the nurse at each visit?

 6. According to Box 15-2 in the textbook, what are some good sources of iron that you could instruct Maggie Gardner to add to her diet?

7. Maggie Gardner is not on iron supplementation at this time; however, list three things that you could teach her about iron supplementation. (*Hint*: See page 307 of your textbook.)

Exercise 2

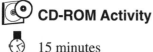 **CD-ROM Activity**

15 minutes

- Sign in to work at Pacific View Regional Hospital on the Obstetrics Floor for Period of Care 3. (*Note*: If you are already in the virtual hospital from a previous exercise, click on **Leave the Floor** and then **Restart the Program** to get to the sign-in window.)
- From the Patient List select Maggie Gardner (Room 204).
- Click on **Go to Nurses' Station**.
- Click on **Chart** and then on **204**.
- Click on **Diagnostic Reports**.

Review information regarding ultrasounds on page 325 in the textbook.

1. List three things that ultrasounds are used for during the first trimester.

2. List three things that ultrasounds are used for during the second and third trimester.

3. What are two forms of ultrasound? When are they used?

4. What type of ultrasound is Maggie Gardner having?

5. Based on the ultrasound findings, how large is her baby?

6. List three abnormalities found on the ultrasound in regard to the placenta.

7. What is the impression from Maggie Gardner's ultrasound in terms of the fetus and the placenta?

8. What are the recommendations regarding follow-up?

Exercise 2

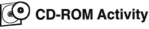 **CD-ROM Activity**

15 minutes

Biophysical profile is another very important assessment tool used with patients who are experiencing a high-risk pregnancy. Review information regarding biophysical profiles on pages 333-335 in the textbook.

1. What five markers are assessed on a biophysical profile? (*Hint:* See Table 16-1 in the textbook.)

2. The amount of amniotic fluid provides information about _____.

3. Normal values for each of the markers listed in question 1 suggest adequate

   _____ and _____.

4. Below, list the markers that are considered acute and those that are considered chronic.

Acute Markers   **Chronic Markers**

 • Sign in to work at Pacific View Regional Hospital on the Obstetrics Floor for Period of Care 3. (*Note*: If you are already in the virtual hospital from a previous exercise, click on **Leave the Floor** and then **Restart the Program** to get to the sign-in window.)

   • From the Patient List, select Kelly Brady.

   • Click on **Go to Nurses' Station**.

   • Click on **Chart** and then on **203**.

   • Click on **Diagnostic Reports**.

5. What is the estimated gestational age of Kelly Brady's fetus?

6. What is the amniotic fluid index as indicated on the report?

7. If Kelly Brady had an abnormally low amount of amniotic fluid, what might this indicate on her report?

8. What is the normal amniotic fluid index value?

9. What is Kelly Brady's score on the biophysical profile?

10. Based on the information you have reviewed in the textbook, what does this score indicate?

LESSON 4

Pain Management for Childbirth

Reading Assignment: Pain Management for Childbirth (Chapter 19)

Patients: Kelly Brady, Room 203
Gabriela Valenzuela, Room 205
Laura Wilson, Room 206

Goal: Demonstrate an understanding of the normal labor and birth process.

Objectives:

- Assess and identify factors that influence pain perception.
- Describe selected nonpharmacologic and pharmacologic measures for pain management during labor and birth.

In this lesson you will compare and contrast the pain management strategies used with three patients during labor and birth.

Exercise 1

 CD-ROM Activity

45 minutes

- Sign in to work at Pacific View Regional Hospital on the Obstetrics Floor for Period of Care 1. (*Note*: If you are already in the virtual hospital from a previous exercise, click on **Leave the Floor** and then **Restart the Program** to get to the sign-in window.)
- From the Patient List, select Laura Wilson.
- Click on **Get Report**.

1. What is Laura Wilson's condition when you assume care for her, according to the change-of-shift report?

65

• Click on **Go to Nurses' Station**.
- Click on Room **206** at the bottom of the screen.
- Read the **Initial Observations**.

2. What is your impression of Laura Wilson's condition?

 • Click on **Patient Care**.
- Click on **Nurse-Client Interactions**.
- Select and view the video titled **0730: Patient Assessment**. (*Note*: If this video is not available, check the virtual clock to see whether enough time has elapsed. The video cannot be viewed before its specified time.)

3. What is Laura Wilson's assessment of her current condition? How does this compare with the information you received from the shift report and the Initial Observations summary?

→ • Click on **Chart** and then on **206**.
- Click on **Nursing Admission**.

4. List Laura Wilson's admission diagnoses. (*Hint:* See page 1 of the Nursing Admission form.)

5. What is your perception of Laura Wilson's behavior? What data did you collect during this exercise that led you to this perception?

6. Think about the following questions and then discuss your ideas with your classmates: Do your personal values and beliefs contribute to your perception of Laura Wilson's behavior? If so, how? What nursing interventions might help to overcome your personal biases when dealing with Laura Wilson?

Read the section on Factors Influencing Pain Response on pages 489-491 in your textbook.

Continue reviewing Laura Wilson's **Nursing Admission** form as needed to answer question 7.

7. Each woman's pain during childbirth is unique and is influenced by a variety of factors. For each factor listed below, explain how that factor influences pain perception (in the middle column). Then, in the right column, list data from Laura Wilson's Nursing Admission that support how that factor might relate to her particular pain perception.

Factor	Typical Effect on Pain Perception	Laura Wilson's Supporting Data
Anxiety		
Previous experience		
Childbirth preparation		
Support		

Exercise 2

 CD-ROM Activity

45 minutes

- Sign in to work at Pacific View Regional Hospital on the Obstetrics Floor for Period of Care 2. (*Note*: If you are already in the virtual hospital from a previous exercise, click on **Leave the Floor** and then **Restart the Program** to get to the sign-in window.)
- From the Patient List, select Gabriela Valenzuela.

Read the sections on Cutaneous Stimulation and Mental Stimulation (pages 422-424) in your textbook.

1. Cutaneous stimulation includes _____, _____,

   _____, and _____. Touch can communicate

   _____, _____, _____, and

   _____.

2. Breathing techniques provide a different focus during contractions, interfering with

   _____. The woman should begin with _____

   patterns and progress to _____ as greater distraction is

   needed. Each contraction begins and ends with a _____. The cleansing

   breath helps the woman release _____ and focus on

   _____, provides _____, and signals her labor partner
   that the contraction is beginning or ending.

Now read the section on Systemic Drugs for Labor on page 430 in your textbook.

- Click on **Get Report**.

3. Is Gabriela Valenzuela in labor at this time? Give a rationale for your answer.

➡ • Click on **Go to Nurses' Station**.
  • Click on Room **205** at the bottom of the screen.
  • Click on **Patient Care**.
  • Click on **Nurse-Client Interactions**.
  • Select and view the video titled **1140: Intervention—Bleeding, Comfort**. (*Note*: If this video is not available, check the virtual clock to see whether enough time has elapsed. The video cannot be viewed before its specified time.)
  • After viewing the video, click on **Chart** and then on **205**.
  • Click on **Nurse's Notes**.
  • Scroll to the entry for 1140 on Wednesday.

4. How is Gabriela Valenzuela tolerating labor at this time?

5. What pain interventions does the nurse implement at this time?

 Read in your textbook about fentanyl in Table 19-1 on page 428 and in the section on Systemic Drugs for Labor on page 430.

6. What is the action of this drug?

Let's begin the process for preparing and administering Gabriela Valenzuela's fentanyl dose.

→ • First, click on **Return to Room 205** and then on **Medication Room**.
  • Next, click on **MAR** and then on tab **205**.
  • Scroll down to the PRN Medication Administration Record for Wednesday.

  7. What is the ordered dose of fentanyl?

→ • Click on **Return to Medication Room**.
  • Click on **Automated System**.
  • Click on **Login**.
  • In box 1, click on **Gabriela Valenzuela, 205**.
  • In box 2, click on **Automated System Drawer A-F**.
  • Click on **Fentanyl citrate**.
  • Click on **Put Medication on Tray**.
  • Click on **Close Drawer**.
  • Click on **View Medication Room**.
  • Click on **Preparation**.
  • Click on **Prepare** and follow the Preparation Wizard prompts to complete preparation of Gabriela Valenzuela's fentanyl dose. When the Wizard stops requesting information, click **Finish**.
  • Click on **Return to Medication Room**.
  • Click on **205** to go to the patient's room.

  8. What additional assessments must be completed before you give Gabriela Valenzuela's medication?

9. Why is it important to check Gabriela Valenzuela's respirations prior to giving the dose of fentanyl?

10. What safety precautions should be in effect for Gabriela Valenzuela after she receives this dose of fentanyl?

→ • Click on **Patient Care** and then **Medication Administration**.
  • Click on **Review Your Medications** and verify the accuracy of your preparation. Click **Return to Room 205**.
  • Next, click the down arrow next to **Select** and choose **Administer**.
  • Follow the Administration Wizard prompts to administer Gabriela Valenzuela's fentanyl dose. (*Note:* Click **Yes** when asked whether to document this administration in the MAR.)
  • When the Wizard stops asking questions, click **Finish**.
  • Still in Gabriela Valenzuela's room, click on **Patient Care**.
  • Click on **Nurse-Client Interactions**.
  • Select and view the video titled: **1155: Evaluation—Comfort Measures**. (*Note*: If this video is not available, check the virtual clock to see whether enough time has elapsed. The video cannot be viewed before its specified time.)

11. How effective were the interventions you identified in question 5?

Read the section on Helping the Woman Use Nonpharmacologic Techniques on page 436 in your textbook.

12. Gabriela Valenzuela is most likely experiencing _____. Other symptoms

of hyperventilation include _____

and _____.

13. What interventions does the nurse suggest to deal with this problem? List other interventions described in your textbook.

 At the end of the 1155 video, Gabriela Valenzuela states that she "doesn't want any needles" in her back. Learn more about this by reading the section on Epidural Block on pages 425-427 in your textbook.

14. What could you tell Gabriela Valenzuela to help her make an informed decision about anesthesia for labor? Below, list advantages and disadvantages of epidural anesthesia.

Advantages   **Disadvantages**

Before leaving this period of care, let's see how you did preparing and administering the patient's medication.

 • Click on **Leave the Floor**.
• Click on **Look at Your Preceptor's Evaluation**.
• Click on **Medication Scorecard** and review the evaluation. How did you do? (*Hint:* For a quick refresher on reading your Medication Scorecard, see page 22 in the **Getting Started** section of this workbook. For a more detailed tour on preparing and administering medications and interpreting your Scorecard, see pages 26-30 and 37-41.)

Exercise 3

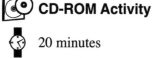 **CD-ROM Activity**

20 minutes

Read the section on General Anesthesia on pages 431-432 in your textbook.

• Sign in to work at Pacific View Regional Hospital on the Obstetrics Floor for Period of Care 4. (*Note*: If you are already in the virtual hospital from a previous exercise, click on **Leave the Floor** and then **Restart the Program** to get to the sign-in window.)
• From the Nurses' Station, click on **Chart** and then on **203** for Kelly Brady's chart.
• Click on **Nurse's Notes**.
• Scroll to the entry for 1730 on Wednesday.

1. Why does the anesthesiologist plan to use general anesthesia during Kelly Brady's cesarean section? (*Hint*: Read the section on Contraindications and Precautions on page 426 in your textbook.)

2. Why is Kelly Brady upset about receiving general anesthesia for her surgery?

• Click on **Physician's Orders**.
 • Review the entry for Wednesday at 1540.

3. What preoperative medications are ordered for Kelly Brady?

 • Click on **Return to Nurses' Station**.
 • Click on the **Drug** icon in the lower left corner of your screen to access the Drug Guide.
 • Use the Search box or the scroll bar to read about each of the drugs you listed in question 3.

4. All of these medications are given preoperatively to help prevent aspiration pneumonia. Using information from the Drug Guide and from the section on General Anesthesia in your textbook, match each of the medications below with the description of how it specifically works to prevent aspiration pneumonia.

_____ Sodium citrate/citric acid (Bicitra)   a. Decreases the production of gastric acid

_____ Metoclopramide (Reglan)   b. Prevents nausea and vomiting and accelerates gastric emptying

_____ Ranitidine (Zantac)

c. Raises the gastric pH to neutralize acidic stomach contents

5. How would you expect general anesthesia to affect Kelly Brady's baby? Why?

The Childbearing Family with Special Needs: Adolescent Pregnancy, Delayed Pregnancy, and Substance Abuse

Reading Assignment: The Childbearing Family with Special Needs
(Chapter 25, pages 593-606)

Patients: Laura Wilson, Room 206
Kelly Brady, Room 203

Goal: Demonstrate an understanding of the special needs of pregnant adolescents, mature primigravidas, and women with substance abuse issues.

Objectives:

* Describe differences in the normal pregnancy changes experienced by adolescent and older mothers.
* Assess and plan care for a substance-abusing woman with a term pregnancy.

In this lesson you will assess and plan care for two pregnant patients with special needs related to maternal age and/or lifestyle (substance abuse).

Exercise 1

CD-ROM Activity

20 minutes

Laura Wilson and Kelly Brady represent age extremes among women of childbearing age. Read the section on Adolescent Pregnancy on pages 593-596 in your textbook.

1. Despite recent decreases, the pregnancy and birth rate for teenagers in the United States

   is _____ when compared with the rate in other developed coun-

   tries. About _____ of teen pregnancies are unintended. Within _____ years,

   _____ of adolescent mothers have another pregnancy.

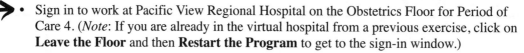 • Sign in to work at Pacific View Regional Hospital on the Obstetrics Floor for Period of Care 4. (*Note*: If you are already in the virtual hospital from a previous exercise, click on **Leave the Floor** and then **Restart the Program** to get to the sign-in window.)

• From the Nurses' Station, click on **Chart** and then on the chart for Room **206**.

• Click on **Nursing Admission**.

2. The table below and on the next page lists several common characteristics of pregnant adolescents, according to your textbook. Based on information found in Nursing Admission, explain how each of these characteristics applies (or does not apply) to Laura WIlson.

Characteristic	Laura Wilson's Supporting Data
Pregnancy is unintended	
No or inadequate prenatal care	
Smoker	
Inadequate weight gain	
Unmarried	

Characteristic	Laura Wilson's Supporting Data
Not ready for emotional, psychologic, and financial responsibilities of parenthood	
High incidence of STDs	

Read the section on Delayed Pregnancy on pages 600-601 in your textbook.

→ • Click on **Return to Nurses' Station**.
   • Click on **Chart** and then on **203** for Kelly Brady's chart.
   • Click on **Nursing Admission**.

3. The table below and on the next page lists several common characteristics of mature primigravidas. Based on the information found in the Nursing Admission, explain how each of these characteristics applies (or does not apply) to Kelly Brady.

Characteristic	Kelly Brady's Supporting Data
Pregnancy delayed to pursue a career or for financial reasons	
Decision to become pregnant made after careful thought	

Characteristic	Kelly Brady's Supporting Data
Usually has financial security, a stable relationship, and personal maturity	
Often adopts health-promoting activities	
Receptive to education on childbearing and/or child-rearing topics. Likely to seek out information from a variety of sources.	
Concerned about complications that may affect the fetus or their own health	

4. Preeclampsia and gestational diabetes occur more frequently in the older gravida.
   a. True
   b. False

5. The risk for multiple birth (twins, triplets, etc.) decreases with advanced maternal age.
   a. True
   b. False

Exercise 2

 CD-ROM Activity

20 minutes

- Sign in to work at Pacific View Regional Hospital on the Obstetrics Floor for Period of Care 2. (*Note*: If you are already in the virtual hospital from a previous exercise, click on **Leave the Floor** and then **Restart the Program** to get to the sign-in window.)
- From the Patient List, select Laura Wilson.
- Click on **Go to Nurses' Station**.
- Click on **Chart** and then on the chart for Room **206**.
- Click on **Nursing Admission**.

1. Based on your review of the Nursing Admission, complete the table below by documenting Laura Wilson's use of alcohol and recreational drugs.

Substance	Reported Use
Tobacco	
Alcohol	
Marijuana	
Crack cocaine	

 Read about the maternal and fetal effects of tobacco, alcohol, marijuana, and cocaine in the Substance Abuse section on pages 601-604 in your textbook.

2. For each pregnancy-related risk listed in the table below, place an X under the substance(s) thought to be associated with that risk.

Maternal or Fetal Effect	Tobacco	Alcohol	Marijuana	Cocaine
Spontaneous abortion				
Premature rupture of membranes				
Preterm labor				
Decreased placental perfusion				
Abruptio placentae				
Fetal alcohol syndrome (FAS)				
Fetal alcohol effects (FAE)				
Hypertension				
Fetal demise				
Anemia				
Inadequate maternal weight gain				
Intrauterine growth restriction (IUGR)				

→
- Click on **Return to Nurses' Station**.
- Click on **206** at the bottom of the screen.
- Click on **Patient Care** and then on **Nurse-Client Interactions**.
- Select and view the video titled **1115: Teaching—Effects of Drug Use**. (*Note*: If this video is not available, check the virtual clock to see whether enough time has elapsed. The video cannot be viewed before its specified time.)

3. Does Laura Wilson consider herself to be addicted? Support your answer with comments from the video.

4. How does Laura Wilson think her drug use will affect her baby?

5. According to the nurse in the video, how might Laura Wilson's drug use affect the baby?

 Read the section on Interventions on page 605 in your textbook.

6. Assume that you are the nurse caring for Laura Wilson today. Which interventions would be most appropriate to deal with Laura Wilson's drug use at this time?

_____ Talk with Laura Wilson in a manner that conveys caring and concern.

_____ Urge Laura Wilson to begin a drug treatment program today.

_____ Explain to Laura Wilson that she may lose custody of her baby if her drug use continues.

_____ Involve other members of the health care team in Laura Wilson's care.

7. Explain your choice(s) in question 6.

The Childbearing Family with Special Needs: Pregnancy Loss and Intimate Partner Violence

/◯⑦✑ **Reading Assignment:** Childbearing Family with Special Needs (Chapter 25)

Patients: Stacey Crider, Room 202
Maggie Gardner, Room 204

Goals: Demonstrate an understanding of the grieving process and how it relates to coping with a current pregnancy.
To identify patients at risk for intimate partner violence, interventions to assist those at risk, and ways to educate and empower those individuals toward health relationships.

Objectives:

- Identify the various types of loss as they relate to a pregnancy.
- Identify various methods of coping exhibited by patients who have experienced the loss of a newborn.
- Discuss the statistics related to intimate partner violence (IPV).
- List characteristics of battered women.
- Explore the myths and facts regarding IPV.
- Identify the nurse's role in regard to battered women or those involved in IPV.

✐ **Exercise 1**

🕐 **Clinical Preparation: Writing Activity**

📚 15 minutes

Review the information on pages 607-609 in the textbook.

1. Parents may grieve not only the death of a newborn but also the birth of a baby with a

_____ or _____.

2. What emotions do parents experience with multifetal pregnancy loss and the concurrent survival of one or more of the infants? How does this affect the grieving process?

3. What potential problems may a previous pregnancy loss cause in a woman experiencing a subsequent pregnancy?

4. All women and men who undergo a loss receive the support that they need.
   a. True
   b. False

Exercise 2

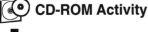 **CD-ROM Activity**

10 minutes

- Sign in to work at Pacific View Regional Hospital on the Obstetrics Floor for Period of Care 4. (*Note*: If you are already in the virtual hospital from a previous exercise, click on **Leave the Floor** and then **Restart the Program** to get to the sign-in window.)
- Click on **Chart** and then on **204** for Maggie Gardner's chart.
- Review the **History and Physical**.

1. How many losses related to pregnancy has Maggie Gardner experienced?

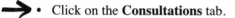 • Click on the **Nursing Admission**.

2. What is the first evidence you find that Maggie Gardner's previous losses are affecting her current pregnancy and care? (*Hint*: Review the first five sections of the Nursing Admission.)

• Click on the **Consultations** tab.

3. To what does Maggie Gardner attribute her inability to have a child?

4. List three therapeutic measures the chaplain can use to assist Maggie Gardner through these feelings as part of her grieving process.

5. What did the chaplain accomplish during his time with Maggie Gardner?

Review page 609 in your textbook.

6. Acknowledging the infant is extremely important in helping the parents work through their loss. What are the rights of the baby that may help the parents through the grieving process?

7. Now that you have read the information regarding the grieving process, let's explore your experiences. Have you ever suffered a loss or taken care of a patient who had just experienced a loss? What emotions did you experience or perceive from that patient? What responses did you communicate to the patient? Were they therapeutic? How might you have handled it differently?

Exercise 3

✏ Clinical Preparation: Writing Activity

🕐 15 minutes

📖 To answer questions 1 through 7, review the information on pages 610-613 in your textbook.

1. Match the statistics on the right to the descriptions of abuse on the left.

_____ The costs associated with IPV—including care, productivity loss	a. 60%
_____ Number of women who are physically assaulted by an intimate partner each year	b. 1%-20%
_____ Percentage of abused women reporting two or more episodes of violence	c. 50%
_____ Percentage of women's homes in which children are also injured	d. 5.8 billion yearly
_____ Estimated percentage of women who are victims of IPV during pregnancy	e. 1.9 million per year
_____ Number of pregnant women affected by IPV	f. 324,000 per year

Women have often been treated inhumanely throughout history. This continues even today. Based on information from the text, please answer true or false to the following questions.

2. IPV may start or increase in frequency and severity during pregnancy and the postpartum period.
   a. True
   b. False

3. Physical abuse during pregnancy may result in maternal or fetal death.
   a. True
   b. False

4. Substance abuse is often associated with physical abuse.
   a. True
   b. False

5. Physical violence is limited to hitting and slapping.
   a. True
   b. False

6. Children who are abused are more like to become abusive as adults compared with children who have never been abused.
   a. True
   b. False

7. An abusive man often attempts to _____ all aspect of the

_____.

Exercise 4

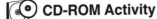 **CD-ROM Activity**

 15 minutes

- Sign in to work at Pacific View Regional Hospital on the Obstetrics Floor for Period of Care 1. (*Note*: If you are already in the virtual hospital from a previous exercise, click on **Leave the Floor** and then **Restart the Program** to get to the sign-in window.)
- From the Patient List, select Dorothy Grant.
- Click on Go to **Nurses' Station**.
- Click on **Chart**.
- Click on the chart for Room **201**.
- Click on the **Nursing Admission** tab.

Review the Nursing Admission for Dorothy Grant's perspective of the abusive relationship that she has experienced. Also review pages 610-611 of the textbook.

1. What is the reality of Dorothy Grant's situation? How does that correlate with the textbook reading?

- Click on **Return to Nurses' Station**.
- Click on Room **201** at the bottom of the screen.
- Click on the **Patient Care**.
- Click on **Nurse-Client Interactions**.
- Select and view the video titled **0810: Monitoring/Patient Support**. (*Note*: If this video is not available, check the virtual clock to see whether enough time has elapsed. The video cannot be viewed before its specified time.)

2. In the video interaction, what does Dorothy Grant say she should do to help prevent the violence?

3. In the video, what are Dorothy Grant's current concerns?

→ • Click on **Go to Nurses' Station**.
 • Click on **Chart**.
 • Click on the chart for Room **201**.
 • Click on **Consultations** and review the Psychiatric Consult and the Social Work Consult.

Review the information regarding the myths and facts about intimate partner violence on page 611 in the textbook. Based on that information and your review of Dorothy Grant's chart, answer the following:

4. Dorothy Grant stays in the relationship because of _____ and

   _____.

5. The percentage of women who are battered during pregnancy is _____.

6. Based on the information provided, in what phase of the abuse cycle is Dorothy Grant?

7. According to the consults, Dorothy Grant has several options. What are some of the options that the social worker and psychiatric heath care provider can offer her or assist her with?

8. Dorothy Grant's husband blames her for the pregnancy.
   a. True
   b. False

9. Dorothy Grant stays in the relationship because likes to be beaten and deliberately provokes the attacks on occasion.
   a. True
   b. False

Exercise 5

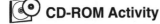 **CD-ROM Activity**

10 minutes

- Sign in to work at Pacific View Regional Hospital on the Obstetrics Floor for Period of Care 4. (*Note*: If you are already in the virtual hospital from a previous exercise, click on **Leave the Floor** and then **Restart the Program** to get to the sign-in window.)
- From the Nurses' Station, click on **Kardex** and then on tab **201** to review Dorothy Grant's record.

1. What action was initiated on Wednesday to protect Dorothy Grant from her husband?

2. What care plan diagnoses are appropriate for this patient's current life situation?

3. What other disciplines have been contacted or consulted to ensure continuity of care for Dorothy Grant as it relates to her abuse?

Review pages 611-612 in your textbook before answering the following questions.

4. As a nurse caring for Dorothy Grant, what is your responsibility for reporting IPV?

5. What are the reporting requirements of the state in which you practice?

6. What are the resources available in your area for women who have experienced intimate partner violence?

The Pregnant Woman with Complications: Hemorrhagic Conditions of Late Pregnancy

Reading Assignment: The Pregnant Woman with Complications
(Chapter 26, pages 624-630)

Patient: Gabriela Valenzuela, Room 205

Goal: Demonstrate an understanding of the identification and management of selected hemorrhagic complications of pregnancy.

Objectives:

- Identify appropriate interventions for managing abruptio placenta.
- Differentiate between the symptoms related to an abruptio placenta and those related to a placenta previa.
- Plan and evaluate essential patient education during the acute phase of diagnosis.

Exercise 1

CD-ROM Activity

45 minutes

- Sign in to work at Pacific View Regional Hospital on the Obstetrics Floor for Period of Care 1. (*Note*: If you are already in the virtual hospital from a previous exercise, click on **Leave the Floor** and then **Restart the Program** to get to the sign-in window.)
- From the Patient List, select Gabriela Valenzuela.
- Click on **Go to Nurses' Station**.
- Click on **Chart** and then on **205**.
- Click on **Emergency Department**.

1. What transpired that brought Gabriela Valenzuela to the ED? How long had she waited to actually come to the ED? What was the deciding factor in her coming to the ED?

 Read about the incidence and etiology of abruptio placenta in your textbook on page 625.

2. Other than a motor vehicle accident, what could result in or increase the risk for having an abruptio placenta?

 3. Differential diagnosis is very important when you are confronted with clinical manifestations that could be evidence of more than one process. Based on the information on pages 624-626 in your textbook, compare and contrast abruptio placenta and placenta previa.

Characteristic/Complication	Abruptio Placenta	Placenta Previa
Bleeding		
Shock complication		
Coagulopathy (DIC)		

Characteristic/Complication	Abruptio Placenta	Placenta Previa
Uterine tonicity		
Tenderness/pain		
Placenta findings		
Fetal effects		

4. Based on your review of the ED Record, what type of abruption does Gabriela Valenzuela have? Provide supporting documentation from your textbook reading. (*Hint*: Review Figure 26-5 on page 626 in your textbook.)

- Click on **Return to Nurses' Station**.
- Click on **205** to go to the patient's room.
- Click on the **Patient Care**.
- Click on **Nurse-Client Interactions**.
- Select and view the video titled **0740: Patient Teaching—Fetal Monitoring**. (*Note*: If this video is not available, check the virtual clock to see whether enough time has elapsed. The video cannot be viewed before its specified time.)

5. Once Gabriela Valenzuela is admitted to the floor, what are her and her husband's concerns? What does the nurse include in her teaching to alleviate those concerns?

Gabriela Valenzuela is at increased risk for early delivery as a result of the abdominal trauma she suffered and the subsequent occurrence of a grade 1 abruptio placenta. She is currently manifesting signs and symptoms of early labor. According to the Physician's Orders, she was given a dose of betamethasone, which was to be repeated in 12 hours.

 6. What is the purpose of the administration of betamethasone in this patient's case? (*Hint*: Review information on page 690 of the textbook.)

→ • Click on **MAR** and review the betamethasone dosage to be given to Gabriela Valenzuela.
  • Click on **Return to Room 205**.
  • Click on **Medication Room**.
  • Click on **Unit Dosage**.
  • Click on drawer **205**.
  • Click on **Betamethasone** in the upper left corner of the screen.
  • Click on **Put Medication on Tray**.
  • Click on **Close Drawer**.
  • Click on **View Medication Room**.
  • Click on **Preparation**.
  • Click on **Prepare** and follow the Preparation Wizard's prompts to complete preparation of Gabriela Valenzuela's betamethasone.
  • When the Wizard stops asking questions, click **Finish**.
  • Click on **Return to Medication Room**.
  • Click on **205** to return to the patient's room.
  • Click on **Patient Care**.
  • Click on **Medication Administration**.
  • Click on **Review Your Medications**.
  • Click on the tab marked **Prepared**.

7. According to the text box on the right side of your screen, what is the medication name and dosage that you have prepared for Gabriela Valenzuela?

8. Based on the answer to the previous question, how many mg are you giving to Gabriela Valenzuela? Is this the correct dosage based on the MAR?

- Click on **Return to Room 205**.
- Click on the **Drug** icon in the left-hand corner of the screen.
- To read about betamethasone, either type the drug name in the Search box or scroll through the alphabetic list of medications at the top of the screen.

9. Based on the information provided in the Drug Guide, what is the indication and dosage for pregnant adults?

10. Based on your review of the baseline assessment data in the Drug Guide, what areas need to be assessed in Gabriela Valenzuela's history?

11. Now review the information regarding the administration of this medication. What are three things that need to be taken into consideration when giving this medication in the injection form?

12. What are the five rights of medication administration as they relate to the patient?

You are now ready to complete the medication administration.

→ • Click on **Return to Room 205**.
   • Click on **Check Armband**.
   • Within the purple box under the patient's photo, find **Betamethasone**. Click the down arrow next to **Select** and choose **Administer**.
   • Follow the Medication Wizard's prompts to administer Gabriela Valenzuela's betamethasone. Click **Yes** when asked whether to document the injection in the MAR.
   • When the Wizard stops asking questions, click **Finish**.
   • Now click on **Nurse-Client Interactions**.
   • Select and view the video titled **0805: Patient Teaching—Abruption**. (*Note*: If this video is not available, check the virtual clock to see whether enough time has elapsed. The video cannot be viewed before its specified time.)

13. According to the video, what will help increase the oxygen supply to the baby and prevent further separation of the placenta?

→ • Click on **Leave the Floor**.
   • Click on **Look at Your Preceptor's Evaluation**.
   • Click on **Medication Scorecard** and review the evaluation. How did you do? (*Hint:* For a quick refresher on reading your Medication Scorecard, see page 22 in the **Getting Started** section of this workbook. For a more detailed tour on preparing and administering medications and interpreting your Scorecard, see pages 26-30 and 37-41.)

Exercise 2

 CD-ROM Activity

30 minutes

- Sign in to work at Pacific View Regional Hospital on the Obstetrics Floor for Period of Care 2. (*Note*: If you are already in the virtual hospital from a previous exercise, click on **Leave the Floor** and then **Restart the Program** to get to the sign-in window.)
- From the Patient List, select Gabriela Valenzuela.
- Click on **Go to Nurses' Station**.
- Click on **Chart**.
- Click on the chart for Room **205**.
- Click on **Diagnostic Reports**.

Gabriela Valenzuela had an ultrasound done on Tuesday to determine the source of the bleeding.

1. What were the findings on the ultrasound?

 - Click on the **Laboratory Reports**.

2. What were Gabriela Valenzuela's hemoglobin and hematocrit levels on Tuesday? How do these findings compare with Wednesday's report? Has there been a significant change?

 3. According to the textbook information, the hematocrit level needs to be maintained above

_____. (*Hint:* See page 657 in the textbook.)

Review the Critical to Remember Box on page 626 in the textbook.

4. What clinical manifestations would indicate a worsening in the condition of either the patient or the fetus?

➡ • Click on **Return to Nurses' Station**.
 • Click on **EPR**.
 • Click on **Login**.
 • Select **205** in the Patient box and **Vital Signs** in the Category box.
 • Using the blue forward and backward arrows, scroll to review the vital signs data over the last 12 hours.

5. From 0000 Wednesday until 1200 Wednesday, would you consider Gabriela Valenzuela's condition stable or unstable? State the rationale for your answer.

➡ • Click on **Exit EPR**
 • Click on **205** at the bottom of the screen.
 • Click on **Patient Care**.
 • Click on **Nurse-Client Interactions**.
 • Select and view the video titled **1140: Intervention—Bleeding, Comfort**. Take notes as you watch and listen. (*Note*: If this video is not available, check the virtual clock to see whether enough time has elapsed. The video cannot be viewed before its specified time.)

6. What happened to elicit this interaction? (*Hint*: Review the Nurse's Notes for Wednesday 1140.)

7. What actions did the nurse take during the video?

Exercise 3

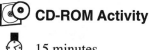 **CD-ROM Activity**

15 minutes

- Sign in to work at Pacific View Regional Hospital on the Obstetrics Floor for Period of Care 3. (*Note*: If you are already in the virtual hospital from a previous exercise, click on **Leave the Floor** and then **Restart the Program** to get to the sign-in window.)
- From the Patient List, select Gabriela Valenzuela.
- Click on **Go to Nurses' Station**.
- Click on **Kardex** and then on tab **205**.

1. What problem areas have been identified by the nurse related to Gabriela Valenzuela's diagnosis?

2. What is the focus of the outcomes related to the problems you listed in question 1?

3. Using correct NANDA nursing diagnosis terminology, list four possible nursing diagnoses appropriate for Gabriela Valenzuela at this time.

• Click on **Return to Nurses' Station**.
• Click on **Chart**.
• Click on the chart for Room **205**.
• Click on **Patient Education**.

4. According to the Patient Education sheet in Gabriela Valenzuela's chart, what are the educational goals related to the patient's diagnosis?

• Click on **Nurse's Notes**.

5. What education has been completed by the nurses through Period of Care 3? Include the times and topics discussed.

6. What are some barriers to learning that the nurse may confront with this patient?

7. How can the nurse overcome each of these?

The Pregnant Woman with Complications: Hypertension During Pregnancy

Reading Assignment: The Pregnant Woman with Complications
(Chapter 26, pages 631-641)

Patient: Kelly Brady, Room 203

Goal: Demonstrate an understanding of the identification and management of severe preeclampsia.

Objectives:

- Assess and identify signs and symptoms present in the patient with severe preeclampsia.
- Explain how common signs and symptoms present in the patient with severe preeclampsia relate to the underlying pathophysiology of this disease.
- Identify the patient who has developed HELLP syndrome.
- Describe routine nursing care for the patient with severe preeclampsia who is receiving magnesium sulfate.

In this lesson you will assess and plan care for a patient with severe preeclampsia who then develops HELLP syndrome and delivers at 26 2/7 weeks gestation.

Exercise 1

CD-ROM Activity

20 minutes

- Sign in to work at Pacific View Regional Hospital on the Obstetrics Floor for Period of Care 3. (*Note*: If you are already in the virtual hospital from a previous exercise, click on **Leave the Floor** and then **Restart the Program** to get to the sign-in window.)
- From the Patient List, select Kelly Brady.
- Click on **Go to Nurses' Station**.
- Click on **Chart** and then on the chart for Room **203**.
- Click on **History and Physical**.

1. What was Kelly Brady's admission diagnosis?

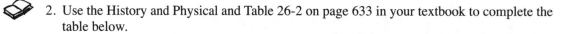 2. Use the History and Physical and Table 26-2 on page 633 in your textbook to complete the table below.

Sign/Symptom	Mild Preeclampsia	Severe Preeclampsia	Kelly Brady on Admission
Systolic blood pressure			
Diastolic blood pressure			
Proteinuria			
Headache (severe, unrelenting, not attributable to other cause)			
Visual disturbances (spots or "sparkles"; temporary blindness; photophobia)			
Right upper quadrant or epigastric pain			

➔ • Click on **Physician's Orders** and find the admitting physician's orders on Tuesday at 1030.

    3. What tests and/or procedures did Kelly Brady's physician order to confirm the diagnosis of severe preeclampsia?

➔ • Click on **Physician's Notes**.
 • Scroll to the note for Wednesday 0730.

    4. What subjective and objective data are recorded here that would support the diagnosis of severe preeclampsia?

Kelly Brady's 24-hour urine collection was completed and sent to the lab at 1230.

➔ • Click on **Laboratory Reports**.
 • Scroll to find the Wednesday 1230 results.

    5. Below, record the results of Kelly Brady's 24-hour urine collection.

Exercise 2

 CD-ROM Activity

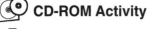 20 minutes

• Sign in to work at Pacific View Regional Hospital on the Obstetrics Floor for Period of Care 1. (*Note*: If you are already in the virtual hospital from a previous exercise, click on **Leave the Floor** and then **Restart the Program** to get to the sign-in window.)
• From the Patient List, select Kelly Brady.
• Click on **Go to Nurses' Station**.
• Click on **203** at the bottom of the screen to go to the patient's room.
• Click on **Take Vital Signs**.

1. Record Kelly Brady's vital signs for 0730 below.

➡ • Now click on **Patient Care**. To perform a focused assessment, select the various body areas (yellow boxes) and system subcategories (green boxes) as listed in question 2.

2. Record your findings from the focused assessment of Kelly Brady in the table below.

Assessment Area	Kelly Brady's Findings
Head & Neck Sensory	
Neurologic	
Chest Respiratory	
Abdomen Gastrointestinal	
Lower Extremities Neurologic	

Read pages 375-376 in your textbook; then answer questions 3 and 4.

3. Preeclampsia is a result of _____ to all body organs as a result

of _____ .

4. Match each of the signs or symptoms below with the preeclampsia-associated pathology it indicates. (*Note:* Some letters will be used more than once.)

_____ Blurred vision/blind spots

_____ Headache

_____ Epigastric pain

_____ Hyperreflexia

_____ Elevated blood pressure

_____ Proteinuria/oliguria

a. Generalized vasoconstriction

b. Glomerular damage

c. Vasoconstriction of cerebral vessels; arterial vasospasm

d. Hepatic edema and subcapsular hemorrhage; hemorrhagic necrosis

Exercise 3

 CD-ROM Activity

30 minutes

- Sign in to work at Pacific View Regional Hospital on the Obstetrics Floor for Period of Care 3. (*Note*: If you are already in the virtual hospital from a previous exercise, click on **Leave the Floor** and then **Restart the Program** to get to the sign-in window.)
- From the Patient List, select Kelly Brady.
- Click on **Go to Nurses' Station**.

Read about HELLP syndrome on page 641 in your textbook.

1. Why do you think Kelly Brady had blood drawn at 1230 for an AST measurement and a platelet count?

→ • Click on **Chart** and then on the chart for Room **203**.
- Click on **Laboratory Reports**.
- Scroll to the report for Wednesday 1230 to locate the results of these tests.

2. Complete the table below based on your review of the Laboratory Reports and your text-book.

Test	Wed 1230 Result	Value in HELLP
Platelet count		
AST		

➤ • Click on **Return to Nurses' Station**.
   • Click on **Patient List**.
   • In the far-right column click on **Get Report** for Kelly Brady.

3. Why has Kelly Brady been transferred to labor and delivery?

4. About half of women with HELLP syndrome also have _____,

   although _____ may be absent. HELLP syndrome consists of intra-

   vascular _____, _____ enzymes, and

   _____ count. The prominent symptom of HELLP syndrome is

   _____.

   Other signs and symptoms include _____, _____, and

   _____.

➤ • Click on **Return to Patient List** and then on **Return to Nurses' Station.**
   • Click on **Chart** and then on **203**.
   • Click on **Physician's Notes**.
   • Scroll to the note for Wednesday 1530.

5. What is the physician's plan of care for Kelly Brady, in light of the HELLP syndrome diag-nosis?

Assume that you will be the nurse caring for Kelly Brady after her surgery while she is receiving magnesium sulfate. Read about this medication on pages 634-635 in your textbook and then answer question 6.

6. All of the assessments/interventions listed below are part of routine nursing care for a patient with severe preeclampsia. Place an X beside the activities that are performed specifically to assess for magnesium toxicity.

_____ Measure/record urine output.

_____ Measure proteinuria using urine dipstick.

_____ Monitor liver enzyme levels and platelet count.

_____ Monitor for headache, visual disturbances, and epigastric pain.

_____ Assess for decreased level of consciousness.

_____ Assess DTRs.

_____ Weigh daily to assess for edema

_____ Monitor vital signs, especially respiratory rate.

_____ Dim room lights and maintain a quiet environment.

The Pregnant Woman with Complications: Gestational Diabetes Mellitus

Reading Assignment: The Pregnant Woman with Complications
(Chapter 26, pages 644-654)

Patient: Stacey Crider, Room 202

Goal: Demonstrate an understanding of the identification and management of gestational diabetes mellitus (GDM).

Objectives:

- Identify appropriate interventions for controlling hyperglycemia in a patient with gestational diabetes mellitus (GDM).
- Correctly administer insulin to a patient with GDM.
- Plan and evaluate essential patient teaching for a patient with GDM.

In this lesson you will describe, plan, and evaluate the care of a patient with gestational diabetes.

Exercise 1

CD-ROM Activity

 30 minutes

- Sign in to work at Pacific View Regional Hospital on the Obstetrics Floor for Period of Care 2. (*Note*: If you are already in the virtual hospital from a previous exercise, click on **Leave the Floor** and then **Restart the Program** to get to the sign-in window.)
- From the Patient List, select Stacey Crider.
- Click on **Go to Nurses' Station**.
- Click on **Chart** and then on the chart for Room **202**.
- Click on **History and Physical**.

1. When was Stacey Crider's GDM diagnosed? How has it been managed thus far?

 2. Read about risk factors for GDM on page 650 in your textbook. List these factors below.

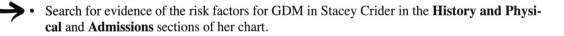 • Search for evidence of the risk factors for GDM in Stacey Crider in the **History and Physical** and **Admissions** sections of her chart.

3. Which risk factors for GDM are present in Stacey Crider?

4. What does Stacey Crider's physician suspect is the cause of her poorly controlled blood glucose levels? (*Hint*: See Impression at the end of the History and Physical.)

• Click on **Physician's Orders**.

5. Look at Stacey Crider's admission orders. Write down the orders that are related to GDM.

 6. Why did Stacey Crider's physician order a hemoglobin A1C test as part of her admission labs? (*Hint*: See page 333 in your textbook.)

On admission, Stacey Crider was in preterm labor. This was treated with magnesium sulfate tocolysis. She was also given a course of betamethasone.

 • Click on **Return to Nurses' Station**.
• Click on the **Drug** icon in the lower left corner of the screen.
• Use the Search box or the scroll bar to find the entry for betamethasone.

7. How might betamethasone affect Stacey Crider's GDM?

• Click on **Return to Nurses' Station**.
• Click on **Chart** and then on **202**.
• Click on **Physician's Notes**.
• Scroll to the note for Tuesday at 0700.

8. How does Stacey Crider's physician plan to deal with these potential medication effects?

Stacey Crider's other admission diagnosis is bacterial vaginosis (BV).

→ • Click on **Return to Nurses' Station**.
 • Click on **202** at the bottom of your screen.
 • Click on **Patient Care** and then on **Nurse-Client Interactions**.
 • Select and view the video titled **1115: Teaching—Diet, Infection**. (*Note*: If this video is not available, check the virtual clock to see whether enough time has elapsed. The video cannot be viewed before its specified time.)

9. What is the relationship between Stacey Crider's bacterial vaginosis infection and her GDM?

Exercise 2

 CD-ROM Activity

⏱ 20 minutes

 • Sign in to work at Pacific View Regional Hospital on the Obstetrics Floor for Period of Care 1. (*Note*: If you are already in the virtual hospital from a previous exercise, click on **Leave the Floor** and then **Restart the Program** to get to the sign-in window.)
 • From the Patient List, select Stacey Crider.
 • Click on **Go to Nurses' Station**.
 • Click on the **Drug** icon in the lower left corner.

Stacey Crider needs her insulin so that she can eat breakfast. Recall that she receives lispro insulin prior to each meal and NPH insulin at bedtime. Read about the different types of insulin in the Drug Guide.

1. Use the information found in the Pharmacokinetics section under the entry for insulin in the Drug Guide to complete the table below.

Type of Insulin	Onset of Action	Peak	Duration
Lispro			
NPH			

Read about proper insulin injection technique in your textbook on page 653.

- Click on **EPR** and then on **Login**.
- Select **202** from the Patient drop-down menu. Select **Vital Signs** in the Category box.
- Look at the vital sign assessment documented on Wednesday at 0700.

2. What was Stacey Crider's blood glucose?

- Click on **Exit EPR**.
- Click on **MAR**.
- Click on tab **202**.

3. What is Stacey Crider's prescribed insulin dosage?

- Click on **Return to Nurses' Station**.
- Click on **Chart**.
- Click on **202**.
- Click on **Physician's Orders**.
- Scroll to the orders for Tuesday at 1900.

4. How much insulin should Stacey Crider receive? Why?

→ • Click on **Return to Nurses' Station**.
 • Click on **Medication Room**.
 • Click on **Unit Dosage**.
 • Click on drawer **202**.
 • Click on **Insulin Lispro**.
 • Click on **Put Medication on Tray**.
 • Click on **Close Drawer**.
 • Click on **View Medication Room**.
 • Click on **Preparation**.
 • Click on **Prepare** and follow the prompts to complete preparation of Stacey Crider's lispro insulin dose.
 • Click on **Return to Medication Room**.

You are almost ready to give Stacey Crider's insulin injection. However, before you do . . .

5. Considering lispro insulin's rapid onset of action, what else should you check before giving Stacey Crider her injection?

Now you're ready!

→ • Click on Room **202**.
 • Click on **Check Armband**.
 • Click on **Patient Care**.
 • Click on **Medication Administration**.
 • **Insulin Lispro** should be listed on the left side of your screen. Click on the down arrow next to **Select** and choose **Administer**.
 • Follow the prompts to administer Stacey Crider's insulin injection. Indicate **Yes** to document the injection in the MAR.
 • Click on **Leave the Floor**.
 • Click on **Look at Your Preceptor's Evaluation**.
 • Click on **Medication Scorecard**. How did you do?

Exercise 3

 CD-ROM Activity

20 minutes

- Sign in to work at Pacific View Regional Hospital on the Obstetrics Floor for Period of Care 3. (*Note*: If you are already in the virtual hospital from a previous exercise, click on **Leave the Floor** and then **Restart the Program** to get to the sign-in window.)
- From the Patient List, select Stacey Crider.
- Click on **Go to Nurses' Station**.
- Click on **Chart** and then on the chart for Room **202**.
- Click on **Patient Education**.

Stacey Crider will likely be discharged home soon. Review her Patient Education record to determine her learning needs in relation to GDM.

1. List the educational goals for Stacey Crider regarding GDM.

Read the section on Nursing Care: The Pregnant Woman with Diabetes Mellitus on pages 652-654 in your textbook.

2. Which of Stacey Crider's educational goals would apply to all women with GDM?

3. Which of Stacey Crider's educational goals would *not* apply to all women with GDM? Support your answer.

• Click on **Nurse's Notes** and scroll to the note for 0600 Wednesday.

4. How did the nurse describe Stacey Crider's ability to give her own insulin injection at that time?

 • Click again on **Patient Education**.

5. What teaching has already been done with this patient on Wednesday in regard to GDM?

• Click on **Nurse's Notes** and scroll to the note for 1200 Wednesday.

6. Do you think today's initial teaching on insulin administration was effective? Support your answer using objective documentation from the nurse's note.

Use the information you have obtained from the Patient Education form and the Nurse's Notes to answer the following questions.

7. Stacey Crider needs to know all of the following information. Which topic(s) would you choose to work on with her during this period of care?

_____ Verbalize appropriate food choices and portions.

_____ Demonstrate good technique when administering insulin.

_____ Demonstrate good technique with self-monitoring of blood glucose.

_____ Recognize hyper- and hypoglycemia and how to treat each.

8. Give a rationale for your answer to question 7.

9. Which topic do you think Stacey Crider would choose to work on during this period of care?

_____   Verbalize appropriate food choices and portions.

_____   Demonstrate good technique when administering insulin.

_____   Demonstrate good technique with self-monitoring of blood glucose.

_____   Recognize hyper- and hypoglycemia and how to treat each.

10. Give a rationale for your answer to question 9.

Read the section on Risk Factors for Gestational Diabetes Mellitus on page 650 in your textbook. Stacey Crider has a significant risk for developing glucose intolerance later in life.

11. What advice would you give Stacey Crider to reduce this risk?

12. Because she has had GDM with this pregnancy, what medical follow-up would you advise for Stacey Crider after her baby is born? Why?

13. Do you believe Stacey Crider's GDM might affect her child? What advice would you give Stacey Crider regarding medical follow-up for her baby?

The Pregnant Woman with Complications: Cardiac Disease/Anemia/Lupus

Reading Assignment: The Pregnant Woman with Complications
(Chapter 26, pages 654-659)

Patients: Maggie Gardner, Room 204
Gabriela Valenzuela, Room 205

Goal: Demonstrate an understanding of the identification and management of selected medical-surgical problems in pregnancy.

Objectives:

- Identify appropriate interventions for managing selected medical-surgical problems in pregnancy.
- Plan and evaluate essential patient education during the acute phase of diagnosis.

Exercise 1

CD-ROM Activity

 10 minutes

- Sign in to work at Pacific View Regional Hospital on the Obstetrics Floor for Period of Care 1. (*Note*: If you are already in the virtual hospital from a previous exercise, click on **Leave the Floor** and then **Restart the Program** to get to the sign-in window.)
- From the Patient List, select Gabriela Valenzuela.
- Click on **Go to Nurses' Station**.
- Click on **Chart** and then on the chart for Room **205**.
- Click on **History and Physical**.

Review material regarding cardiac problems during pregnancy on pages 654-657 in the textbook.

1. According to the textbook, 2%-3% of pregnancies are complicated by heart disease. In the History and Physical for Gabriela Valenzuela, what does the physician note as her cardiac problem?

2. Mitral valve disease is one of the most common causes of cardiac disease in pregnant women.
   a. True
   b. False

3. According to the History and Physical, what cardiac symptoms does Gabriela Valenzuela exhibit now that she is pregnant?

4. Based on your textbook reading, why do pregnant women with cardiac disorders have problems during their pregnancy?

5. What abnormal assessment finding is noted in the History and Physical that would be associated with Gabriela Valenzuela's cardiac disorder?

Exercise 2

 CD-ROM Activity

 20 minutes

 Autoimmune disorders encompass a wide variety of disorders that can be disruptive to the pregnancy process. Maggie Gardner has been admitted to rule out lupus. The following activities will explore the various aspects of this autoimmune disorder. Review the information regarding systemic lupus erythematosus (SLE) on page 659 in your textbook.

- Sign in to work at Pacific View Regional Hospital on the Obstetrics Floor for Period of Care 1. (*Note*: If you are already in the virtual hospital from a previous exercise, click on **Leave the Floor** and then **Restart the Program** to get to the sign-in window.)
- From the Patient List, select Maggie Gardner.
- Click on **Go to Nurses' Station**.
- Click on **Chart** and then on the chart for Room **204**.
- Click on **History and Physical**.

1. Based on Maggie Gardner's History and Physical, what information would correlate to a diagnosis of SLE?

 2. According to the textbook, what is most often the presenting symptom of this disease during pregnancy?

→ • Click on **Return to Nurses' Station**.
- Click on Room **204** at the bottom of the screen.
- Click on **Patient Care**.
- Click on **Physical Assessment**.
- Click on the various body areas (yellow boxes) and system subcategories (green boxes) to perform a head-to-toe assessment of Maggie Gardner.

3. Based on your head-to-toe assessment, list four abnormal findings that are related to Maggie Gardner's diagnosis.

 • Click on **Chart** and then on **204**.
  • Click on **Patient Education**.

4. Based on your physical assessment, the information from the Patient Education section of the chart, and the fact that this is a new diagnosis for the patient, list three areas of teaching that need to be completed with this patient.

Exercise 3

 CD-ROM Activity

35 minutes

- Sign in to work at Pacific View Regional Hospital on the Obstetrics Floor for Period of Care 3. (*Note*: If you are already in the virtual hospital from a previous exercise, click on **Leave the Floor** and then **Restart the Program** to get to the sign-in window.)
- From the Patient List, select Maggie Gardner.
- Click on **Go to Nurses' Station**.
- Click on **Chart**.
- Click on the chart for Room **204**.
- Click on the **Consultations** tab.
- Review the Rheumatology Consult.

1. List four things noted in the rheumatologist's impressions regarding specific findings that are associated with a diagnosis of SLE for Maggie Gardner.

 • Click on **Diagnostic Reports**.

2. Maggie Gardner had an ultrasound done prior to the consultation with the rheumatologist. What were the findings as they relate to SLE? What were the follow-up recommendations? (*Hint*: See Impressions section.)

3. What is the rheumatologist's plan regarding laboratory/diagnostics to gain a definitive diagnosis?

4. According to the Rheumatology Consult, what is the plan regarding medications (immediate need)?

- Click on **Return to Nurses' Station**.
- Click on the **Drug** icon in the lower left corner of the screen.
- Find the Drug Guide profile of prednisone. (*Hint:* You can type the drug name in the Search box or scroll through the alphabetic list of drugs at the top of the screen.)

5. What does Maggie Gardner need to be taught regarding this medication?

- Click on **Return to Nurses' Station**.
- Click on Room **204**.
- Click on **Patient Care**.
- Click on **Nurse-Client Interactions**.
- Select and view the video titled **1530: Disease Management**. (*Note:* If this video is not available, check the virtual clock to see whether enough time has elapsed. The video cannot be viewed before its specified time.)

6. During this video clip, the nurse provides Maggie Gardner with information regarding her disease. What two things does the nurse note that are important aspects of the patient's disease management during pregnancy?

7. What medication, ordered by the rheumatologist, will assist in the blood flow to the placenta? How?

8. What key component does the nurse identify for Maggie Gardner that will assist in maintaining a healthy pregnancy?

9. What excuse does Maggie Gardner give for not keeping previous doctor's appointments? (*Hint:* This information is also found in the Nursing Admission in the chart.)

Exercise 4

 CD-ROM Activity

15 minutes

- Sign in to work at Pacific View Regional Hospital on the Obstetrics Floor for Period of Care 4. (*Note*: If you are already in the virtual hospital from a previous exercise, click on **Leave the Floor** and then **Restart the Program** to get to the sign-in window.)
- From the Nurses' Station, click on **Chart**.
- Click on **204** to open Maggie Gardner's chart.
- Click on **Laboratory Reports**.

1. The results are now available for the following laboratory tests that were ordered during Period of Care 2. What are the findings?

Laboratory Test	Result
C3	
C4	
CH50	
RPR	
ANA titer	
Anticardiolipin	
Anti-sm; Anti-DNA; Anti–SSA	
Anti-SSB	
Anti-RVV; Antiphospholipid	

- Click on **Consultations** and review the Rheumatology Consult.

2. The lab findings you recorded in question 1 are definitive for the diagnosis of SLE. According to the textbook and the Rheumatology Consult, what is the plan to manage this disease once Maggie Gardner's baby is delivered?

→ • Click on **Nurse's Notes.**

3. By Period of Care 4, Maggie Gardner has been provided with education regarding various aspects of her disease process, testing, and hospital procedures. Based on your review of the Nurse's Notes for Wednesday, what has she been specifically taught? Include the time each instruction took place.

4. Using correct NANDA nursing diagnosis terminology, write three possible nursing diagnoses for Maggie Gardner.

5. SLE requires long-term management because patients will experience remissions and exacerbations. What step did the rheumatologist take with Maggie Gardner to begin the long-term relationship that will be required to ensure a healthy outcome?

The Pregnant Woman with Complications: Infections During Pregnancy

Reading Assignment: The Pregnant Woman with Complications
(Chapter 26, pages 661-667)

Patients: Gabriela Valenzuela, Room 205
Laura Wilson, Room 206

Goal: Demonstrate an understanding of the identification and management of selected sexually transmitted and other infections in pregnant women.

Objectives:

- Explain the importance of prophylactic Group B streptococcus (GBS) treatment.
- Identify risk factors for acquiring HIV infection.
- Prioritize information to be included in patient teaching related to HIV infection.

In this lesson you will assess and evaluate the care provided to two pregnant women with actual or potential infections that could adversely affect their infants.

Exercise 1

 CD-ROM Activity

15 minutes

- Sign in to work at Pacific View Regional Hospital on the Obstetrics Floor for Period of Care 1. (*Note*: If you are already in the virtual hospital from a previous exercise, click on **Leave the Floor** and then **Restart the Program** to get to the sign-in window.)
- From the Patient List, select Gabriela Valenzuela.
- Click on **Go to Nurses' Station**.
- Click on **Chart** and then on chart for Room **205**.
- Click on **History and Physical** and scroll to the plan at the end of this document.

1. What is the medical plan of care for Gabriela Valenzuela?

2. Is Gabriela Valenzuela known to be positive for Group B streptococcus (GBS)?

Read about Group B streptococcus on pages 666-667 in your textbook; then answer questions 3 through 6.

3. List risk factors for neonatal GBS infection. Which risk factor applies to Gabriela Valenzuela?

4. Since pregnant women with GBS in the vagina are almost always asymptomatic, why does Gabriela Valenzuela need to be treated for this organism?

• Click on **Physician's Orders**.
 • Scroll to the admission orders written Tuesday at 2100.

5. What medication/dosage/frequency will Gabriela Valenzuela receive for Group B strep prophylaxis?

 6. How does this order compare with the treatment regimen recommended in your textbook?

Exercise 2

CD-ROM Activity

35 minutes

• Sign in to work at Pacific View Regional Hospital on the Obstetrics Floor for Period of Care 1. (*Note*: If you are already in the virtual hospital from a previous exercise, click on **Leave the Floor** and then **Restart the Program** to get to the sign-in window.)
• From the Patient List, select Laura Wilson.
• Click on **Go to Nurses' Station**.
• Click on **Chart** and then on chart for Room **206**.
• Click on **Nursing Admission**.

1. What risk factors for acquiring an STI are identified on Laura Wilson's Nursing Admission form?

2. In the United States, homosexual individuals are currently still more likely than heterosexuals to become infected with HIV.
   a. True
   b. False

→ • While still in the chart, click on **Admissions**.

3. In the United States today, HIV infection is spreading most rapidly in the groups listed below. Place an X next to the group(s) to which Laura Wilson belongs.

   _____ a. Women

   _____ b. African American women

   _____ c. Hispanic women

   _____ d. Women who live in the southern United States

→ • Now click again on **Nursing Admission**.

4. What did the admitting nurse document about Laura Wilson's knowledge and acceptance of her HIV diagnosis?

→ • Click on **Return to Nurses' Station** and then on **206** to visit the patient.
 • Click on **Patient Care**.
 • Click on **Nurse-Client Interactions**.
 • Select and view the video titled **0800: Teaching—HIV in Pregnancy**. (*Note*: If this video is not available, check the virtual clock to see whether enough time has elapsed. The video cannot be viewed before its specified time.)

5. Does Laura Wilson appear to be fully aware of the implications of HIV infection? State the rationale for your answer.

6. What coping mechanism is Laura Wilson exhibiting in the video interaction?

→ • Click on **Chart** and then on **206**.
  • Click on **Nursing Admission**.

7. Laura Wilson needs education on all of the following topics. Which would you choose to teach her about at this time?

_____ Safer sex

_____ Medication side effects and importance of compliance

_____ Need for medical follow-up and medication for the baby

_____ Impact of HIV on birth plans

8. Give a rationale for your answer to question 7.

The Woman with an Intrapartum Complication

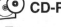 **Reading Assignment:** Nursing Care During Obstetric Procedures
(Chapter 20, pages 454-462)
The Woman with an Intrapartum Complication (Chapter 27)

Patients: Dorothy Grant, Room 201
Stacey Crider, Room 202
Kelly Brady, Room 203
Gabriela Valenzuela, Room 205

Goal: Demonstrate an understanding of the identification and management of selected labor and birth complications.

Objectives:

- Assess and identify signs and symptoms present in the patient with preterm labor.
- Describe appropriate nursing care for the patient in preterm labor.
- Develop a birth plan to meet the needs of the preterm infant.

In this lesson you will compare and contrast the care of four patients, all of whom are treated for preterm labor and/or will deliver preterm infants.

Exercise 1

CD-ROM Activity

20 minutes

- Sign in to work at Pacific View Regional Hospital on the Obstetrics Floor for Period of Care 2. (*Note*: If you are already in the virtual hospital from a previous exercise, click on **Leave the Floor** and then **Restart the Program** to get to the sign-in window.)
- From the Patient List, select Dorothy Grant and Gabriela Valenzuela.
- Click on **Go to Nurses' Station**.
- Click on **Chart** and then on **201** for Dorothy Grant's chart.
- Click on **History and Physical**.

1. Using the information found in the History and Physical section, complete the table below for Dorothy Grant.

Patient	Weeks Gestation	Reason for Admission
Dorothy Grant		

➡ • Click on **Return to Nurses' Station**.
   • Now click again on **Chart**; this time, select **205** for Gabriela Valenzuela's chart.
   • Click on **History and Physical**.

2. Using the information found in the History and Physical section, complete the table below for Gabriela Valenzuela.

Patient	Weeks Gestation	Reason for Admission
Gabriela Valenzuela		

➡ • Click on **Return to Nurses' Station**.
   • Click on **201** at the bottom of the screen to go to Dorothy Grant's room.
   • Click on **Patient Care**.
   • Click on **Physical Assessment**.
   • Click on **Pelvic** and then on **Reproductive**.

3. Complete the table below with the results of Dorothy Grant's initial cervical examination.

Patient	Time	Dilation	Effacement	Station
Dorothy Grant				

→ • Click on **Return to Nurses' Station**.
   • Click on **205** to go to Gabriela Valenzuela's room.
   • Click on **Patient Care**.
   • Click on **Physical Assessment**.
   • Click on **Pelvic** and then on **Reproductive**.

4. Record the results of Gabriela Valenzuela's initial cervical examination in the table below.

Patient	Time	Dilation	Effacement	Station
Gabriela Valenzuela				

Read the definition of preterm labor on page 698 in your textbook. Also consult Table 17-1 on page 355.

5. Preterm labor is defined as the onset of labor after _____

   but before _____.

6. As of Wednesday at 0800, would you consider both these patients to be in preterm labor? Give a rationale for your answer.

Read the section on Tocolytics on pages 686-689 in your textbook to answer the following questions.

7. Match each medication below with the description of how it works as a tocolytic agent. (*Hint:* Letters may be used more than once.)

_____ Magnesium sulfate

_____ Nifedipine (Procardia)

_____ Ritodrine (Yutopar)

_____ Terbutaline (Brethine)

_____ Indomethacin (Indocin)

a. Blocks calcium from entering smooth muscle cells, thus relaxing uterine contractions

b. Inhibits uterine muscle activity as a result of stimulation of beta-adrenergic receptors of the sympathetic nervous system

c. Exact mechanism unclear, but promotes relaxation of smooth muscles

d. Suppresses preterm labor by inhibiting the synthesis of prostaglandins

Exercise 2

 CD-ROM Activity

30 minutes

- Sign in to work at Pacific View Regional Hospital on the Obstetrics Floor for Period of Care 1. (*Note*: If you are already in the virtual hospital from a previous exercise, click on **Leave the Floor** and then **Restart the Program** to get to the sign-in window.)
- From the Patient List, select Stacey Crider.
- Click on **Get Report**.

Stacey Crider was admitted yesterday in preterm labor and given magnesium sulfate. Her other admission diagnoses were bacterial vaginosis and gestational diabetes with poorly controlled blood glucose levels.

1. What is Stacey Crider's current status in regard to preterm labor?

 • Click on **Go to Nurses' Station**.
- Click on **Chart** and then on the chart for Room **202**.
- Click on **Physician's Orders**.
- Scroll to the orders for Wednesday at 0715.

2. Which of these orders relate specifically to Stacey Crider's diagnosis of preterm labor?

→ • Scroll to the orders for Wednesday at 0730.

3. What medication changes are ordered?

 Read the Terbutaline Drug Guide on page 688 in your textbook.

4. Why do you think Stacey Crider's physician changed the orders so quickly?

→ • Click on **Return to Nurses' Station**.
 • Click on **202** at the bottom of the screen.
 • Inside the patient's room, click on **Take Vital Signs**.

5. What are Stacey Crider's current vital signs?

Temperature

Pulse

Respiration

Blood pressure

6. Which of these parameters provides the most important information you would need prior to giving Stacey Crider's nifedipine dose? Why? (*Hint*: Read about nifedipine on page 551 in your textbook.)

Like Dorothy Grant and Kelly Brady, Stacey Crider is also receiving betamethasone.

 Read about Accelerating Fetal Lung Maturity in your textbook on page 689. Also consult the Betamethasone, Dexamethasone Drug Guide on page 690. Then answer the following questions.

7. Why are all three of these patients receiving antenatal glucocorticoid therapy?

8. What other benefit does this class of medication seem to provide for preterm infants?

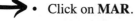 • Click on **MAR**.
  • Click on tab **202**.

9. What is Stacey Crider's prescribed betamethasone dosage?

10. How does this dosage compare with the recommended dosage in your textbook?

→ • Click on **Return to Nurses' Station**.
 • Click on **Medication Room**.
 • Click on **Unit Dosage**.
 • Click on drawer **202**.
 • Click on **Betamethasone**.
 • Click on **Put Medication on Tray**.
 • Click on **Close Drawer**.
 • Click on **View Medication Room**.
 • Click on **Preparation**.
 • Click on **Prepare** and follow the preparation Wizard's prompts to complete preparation of Stacey Crider's betamethasone dose.
 • Click on **Return to Medication Room**.
 • Click on **202** to return to Stacey Crider's room.
 • Click on **Check Armband**.
 • Click on **Check Allergies**.
 • Click on **Patient Care**.
 • Click on **Medication Administration**.
 • Find **Betamethasone** listed on the left side of your screen. To its right, click on the down arrow next to **Select** and choose **Administer**.
 • Follow the Administration Wizard's prompts to administer Stacey Crider's betamethasone injection. Indicate **Yes** to document the injection in the MAR.
 • Click on **Leave the Floor**.
 • Click on **Look at Your Preceptor's Evaluation**.
 • Click on **Medication Scorecard**. How did you do?

Exercise 3

 CD-ROM Activity

 30 minutes

- Sign in to work at Pacific View Regional Hospital on the Obstetrics Floor for Period of Care 4. (*Note*: If you are already in the virtual hospital from a previous exercise, click on **Leave the Floor** and then **Restart the Program** to get to the sign-in window.)
- From the Nurses' Station, click on **Chart**.
- Click on **201** for Dorothy Grant's chart.
- Click on **Nurse's Notes**.
- Scroll to the note for Wednesday 1815.

1. What are the findings from Dorothy Grant's cervical examination at this time?

 • Scroll to the note for Wednesday 1840. It states that Dorothy Grant is being prepped for delivery.

2. If you were the nurse caring for Dorothy Grant during delivery, what special preparations would you make to care for the baby immediately after birth? (*Hint:* Read Teaching What May Occur During a Preterm Birth on page 691 in your textbook.)

→ • Click on **Return to Nurses' Station**.
   • Click again on **Chart**, but this time choose **205** for Gabriela Valenzuela's chart.
   • Click on **Physician's Notes**.
   • Scroll to the note for Wednesday 0800.

   3. What is the anticipated outcome of Gabriela Valenzuela's labor, according to this note?

→ • Scroll to the notes for Wednesday 1415 and 1455.

   4. What preparations have been made during the day for the birth of Gabriela Valenzuela's baby?

 Read the information on cesarean birth found on pages 454-462 in your textbook.

→ • Click on **Return to Nurses' Station**.
   • Once again, click on **Chart**; select **203** for Kelly Brady's chart.
   • Click on **Physician's Notes**.
   • Scroll to the note for Wednesday 1530.

Kelly Brady was admitted yesterday with severe preeclampsia at 26 weeks gestation. Her preeclampsia is now worsening.

5. Why does her physician now recommend immediate delivery?

6. What general risks related to cesarean section does Kelly Brady's physician discuss with her?

7. Because of Kelly Brady's early gestational age (26 weeks), her physician anticipates a classical uterine incision. How will this type of incision affect Kelly Brady's birth options in future pregnancies?

→ • Click on **Physician's Orders**.
  • Scroll to the orders for Wednesday 1540.

8. List the orders to be carried out prior to Kelly Brady's surgery. State the purpose of each.

Order	Purpose

9. Can you think of other common preoperative procedures? List them below. (*Hint*: Refer to a basic Medical-Surgical textbook for ideas if you need help!)

LESSON 13

Medication Administration

Patients: Dorothy Grant, Room 201
Stacey Crider, Room 202
Maggie Gardner, Room 204
Laura Wilson, Room 206

Goal: Correctly administer selected medications to obstetric patients.

Objective:

• Correctly administer selected medications to obstetric patients, observing the Five Rights.

In this lesson you will give medications to selected obstetric patients, observing the Five Rights.

Exercise 1

CD-ROM Activity

30 minutes

Dorothy Grant was admitted at 30 weeks gestation for observation following blunt abdominal trauma (she was kicked in the abdomen). She is bleeding vaginally and may have sustained a placental abruption. Your assignment for this exercise is to give Rho(D) immune globulin to her.

• Sign in to work at Pacific View Regional Hospital on the Obstetrics Floor for Period of Care 2. (*Note*: If you are already in the virtual hospital from a previous exercise, click on **Leave the Floor** and then **Restart the Program** to get to the sign-in window.)
• From the Patient List, select Dorothy Grant.

 Read about Rho(D) immune globulin on page 644 in your textbook.

1. Rho(D) immune globulin is given to prevent _____

in Rh-_____ women who have been exposed to Rh-_____ blood.

Rho(D) immune globulin prevents sensitization by _____

_____.

2. All of the following are reasons that Rho(D) immune globulin might be administered. Place an X next to the reason it has been ordered for Dorothy Grant.

_____ Within 72 hours of giving birth to an Rh-positive infant

_____ Prophylactically at 28 weeks gestation

_____ Following an incident or exposure risk that occurs after 28 weeks gestation

_____ During first trimester of pregnancy following miscarriage or elective abortion or ectopic pregnancy

3. List the information about Dorothy Grant that must be determined before giving her Rho(D) immune globulin.

- Click on **Go to Nurses' Station**.
- Click on **Chart** and then on **201**.
- Click on **Physician's Orders**.
- Scroll to the orders for Wednesday 0730.

4. Write the physician's order for Rho(D) immune globulin.

5. According to your textbook, is this the correct dosage and route? (*Hint:* Read the section on Postpartum Management on page 643 in your textbook.)

- Click on **Laboratory Reports**.
- Locate the results for 0245 Wednesday.
- Scroll down to find the type and screen results.

6. Dorothy Grant's blood type is _____.

7. What additional information do you need? Why? Is that information available?

 • Click on **Return to Nurses' Station**.
- Click on **Medication Room**.
- Click on **Refrigerator**; then click on the refrigerator door to open it.
- Click on **Put Medication on Tray**.
- Click on **Close Door**.
- Click on **View Medication Room**.
- Click on **Preparation**.
- Click on **Prepare** and follow the prompts to complete preparation of this medication.
- Click on **Return to Medication Room**.
- Click on **201** to go to Dorothy Grant's room.
- Click on **Check Armband**.
- Click on **Patient Care**.
- Click on **Medication Administration**.

You are almost ready to give Dorothy Grant's injection. However, before you do . . .

8. Rho(D) immune globulin is often considered a blood product.
   a. True
   b. False

9. Suppose Dorothy Grant tells you that she is a Jehovah's Witness and absolutely refuses to accept blood or blood products. How would you handle the situation?

Now you're ready to administer the medication!

- Click on the down arrow next to **Select**; choose **Administer**.
- Follow the prompts to administer Dorothy Grant's injection. Indicate **Yes** to document the injection in the MAR.
- Click on **Leave the Floor**.
- Click on **Look at Your Preceptor's Evaluation**.
- Click on **Medication Scorecard**. How did you do?

Exercise 2

CD-ROM Activity

20 minutes

- Sign in to work at Pacific View Regional Hospital on the Obstetrics Floor for Period of Care 1. (*Note*: If you are already in the virtual hospital from a previous exercise, click on **Leave the Floor** and then **Restart the Program** to get to the sign-in window.)
- From the Patient List, select Maggie Gardner.
- Click on **Go to Nurses' Station**.
- Click on the **Chart** and then on **204**.
- Click on the **Nursing Admission**.

1. Maggie Gardner verbalizes anxiety repeatedly throughout the Nursing Admission. What is her primary concern? Why? Provide documentation.

2. Maggie Gardner states that before this pregnancy she had a highly adaptive coping mechanism. How does she consider her ability to cope at this point? Why? (*Hint*: See the Coping and Stress Tolerance section in the Nursing Admission.)

➜ • Click on **Physician's Orders**.

   3. What medication has the physician ordered to help Maggie Gardner with her anxiety?

➜ • Click on **Return to Nurses' Station**.
  • Click on the **Drug** icon in the lower-left corner of your screen.
  • Use the Search box or the scroll bar to find the medication you identified in question 3.
  • Review all of the information provided regarding this drug.

   4. What is the drug's mechanism of action?

➜ • Click on **Return to Nurses' Station**.
  • Click on **204** to go to Maggie Gardner's room.
  • Click on **Patient Care**.
  • Click on **Nurse-Client Interactions**.
  • Select and view the video titled **0745: Evaluation—Efficacy of Drugs**. (*Note*: If this video is not available, check the virtual clock to see whether enough time has elapsed. The video cannot be viewed before its specified time.)

   5. According to the nurse, how long will it take for Maggie Gardner to see therapeutic effects? How does this correlate with what you learned in the Teaching Section of the Drug Guide?

Exercise 3

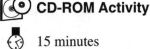 **CD-ROM Activity**

15 minutes

In this exercise, you will administer betamethasone to Stacey Crider, who was admitted to the hospital at 27 weeks gestation in preterm labor.

- Sign in to work at Pacific View Regional Hospital on the Obstetrics Floor for Period of Care 1. (*Note*: If you are already in the virtual hospital from a previous exercise, click on **Leave the Floor** and then **Restart the Program** to get to the sign-in window.)
- From the Patient List, select Stacey Crider.

   1. Before preparing Stacey Crider's betamethasone, what do you need to do first?

 • Click on **Go to Nurses' Station**.
- Click on **Chart** and then on the chart for Room **202**.
- Click on **Physician's Orders**.
- Scroll until you find the order for betamethasone.

   2. After verifying the physician's order, what's your next step?

 • Click on **Return to Nurses' Station**.
- Click on **Medication Room**.
- Click on **Unit Dosage**.
- Click on drawer **202**.
- Click on **Betamethasone**.
- Click on **Put Medication on Tray**.
- Click on **Close Drawer**.
- Click on **View Medication Room**.
- Click on **Preparation**.
- Click on **Prepare** and follow the prompts to complete preparation of Stacey Crider's betamethasone dose.
- Click on **Return to Medication Room**.

3. Now that the medication is prepared, what's your next step?

→ • Click on **202** to go to the patient's room.
  • Click on **Check Armband**.
  • Click on **Check Allergies**.
  • Click on **Patient Care**.
  • Click on **Medication Administration**.
  • Click on the down arrow next to **Select** and choose **Administer**.
  • Follow the prompts to administer Stacey Crider's betamethasone injection.

4. What's the final step in the process?

→ • If you haven't already, indicate **Yes** to document the injection in the MAR.
  • Click on **Leave the Floor**.
  • Click on **Look at Your Preceptor's Evaluation**.
  • Click on **Medication Scorecard**. How did you do?

Exercise 4

CD-ROM Activity

30 minutes

• Sign in to work at Pacific View Regional Hospital on the Obstetrics Floor for Period of Care 1. (*Note*: If you are already in the virtual hospital from a previous exercise, click on **Leave the Floor** and then **Restart the Program** to get to the sign-in window.)
• From the Patient List, select Laura Wilson.
• Click on **Go to Nurses' Station**.
• Click on **MAR**.
• Click on the tab for Room **206**.

1. Laura Wilson's medications for Wednesday include several different types of drugs. In the list below, place an X next to the one that is used to treat her HIV-positive status.

_____ Zidovudine 200 mg po every 8 hours

_____ Prenatal multivitamin 1 tablet po daily

_____ Lactated Ringer's 1000 mL IV continuous

→ • Click on **Return to Nurses' Station**.
   • Click on the **Drug** icon in the lower-left corner of the screen.
   • Using the Search box or the scroll bar, find the drug you identified in question 1.

2. What is the drug's mechanism of action?

3. What is the drug's therapeutic effect?

4. Does this medication cross the placenta, or is it distributed in breast milk?

5. What symptoms/side effects of this medication need to be reported to the physician?

6. How should this medication be taken?

7. Your final assignment is to give Laura Wilson the medication that is due at 0800. During these lessons, we have provided you with the detailed instructions on how to give medications. Now it is time for you to fly solo. Don't forget the Five Rights of medication administration . . . and have fun!! Document below how you did.

If you'd like to get more practice, there are other medications that can be given at the beginning of the first three periods of care. Below is a list of the patients, the medications, the routes of administration, and the administration times you can use. As you practice, be sure to select the correct patient when you sign in. That way, you can get a Medication Scorecard for evaluation after you prepare and administer a medication. (*Remember:* If you need help at any time, refer to pages 22, 26-30, and 37-41 in the **Getting Started** section of this workbook.)

PERIOD OF CARE 1

Room 201, Dorothy Grant

0730/0800

Betamethasone 12 mg IM

Prenatal multivitamin PO

Room 202, Stacey Crider

0800—Prenatal multivitamin PO

Metronidazole 500 mg PO

Betamethasone 12 mg IM

Insulin lispro Sub-Q

Nifedipine 20 mg PO

Room 203, Kelly Brady

0730/0800—Prenatal multivitamin PO

Ferrous sulfate PO

Labetalol hydrochloride 400 mg PO

Nifedipine 10 mg PO

Room 204, Maggie Gardner

0800—Prenatal multivitamin PO

Buspirone hydrochloride 5 mg PO

Room 205, Gabriela Valenzuela

0800—Ampicillin 2 g IV

Betamethasone 12 mg IM

Prenatal multivitamin PO

Room 206, Laura Wilson

0800—Zidovudine 200 mg PO

Prenatal multivitamin PO

PERIOD OF CARE 2

Room 201, Dorothy Grant

1200—Rho(D) immune globulin IM

Room 202, Stacey Crider

1200—Insulin lispro Sub-Q

Room 203, Kelly Brady

1130—Betamethasone 12 mg IM

Room 204, Maggie Gardner

1115—Prednisone 40 mg PO

Aspirin 81 mg PO

PERIOD OF CARE 3

Room 204, Maggie Gardner

1500—Buspirone 5 mg PO

LESSON **14** _____

Caring for An Infant with Bronchiolitis

_____

👓 **Reading Assignment:** Health Promotion for the Infant (Chapter 5, pages 78-101)
Principles and Procedures for Nursing Care of Children
   (Chapter 37, pages 951-952 and 957-960)
The Child with a Respiratory Alteration
   (Chapter 45, pages 1213-1216)

Patient: Carrie Richards, Room 303

Goal: Demonstrate an understanding of nursing care for an infant with bronchiolitis.

Objectives:

• Discuss etiology and pathophysiology of bronchiolitis.
• Relate the effect of an infant's level of growth and development on bronchiolitis.
• Complete a respiratory assessment on an infant and discuss nursing care issues.
• Use the nursing process to develop a nursing care plan for an infant with bronchiolitis.

In this lesson, you will learn and reinforce concepts related to a common respiratory illness in infants. You will apply principles of growth and development in making nursing care decisions. You will be expected to recall/review basic oral and written communication, teaching skills, and family-centered care. Your patient is Carrie Richards, a 3½-month-old who has been admitted to the Pediatric Unit from the Emergency Department. Carrie's medical diagnosis is bronchiolitis. Her mother is with her.

Exercise 1

 Clinical Preparation: Writing Activity

15 minutes

1. Explain the pathophysiology of bronchiolitis.

2. Explain the relationship of respiratory syncitial virus to bronchiolitis.

3. Relate the effect of Carrie's growth and development on her physiologic status.

4. Think about how you would explain a diagnosis of bronchiolitis to Carrie's mother. What information and would you share? How would you present it?

Exercise 2

 CD-ROM Activity

30 minutes

- Sign in to work at Pacific View Regional Hospital on the Pediatrics Floor for Period of Care 1. (*Note:* If you are already in the virtual hospital from a previous exercise, click on **Leave the Floor** and then **Restart the Program** to get to the sign-in window.)
- From the Patient List, select Carrie Richards.
- Click on **Go to Nurses' Station**.
- Click on **Chart** and then on **303** for Carrie's chart.
- Click on **Emergency Department** and review this record.
- Also click and review the **Physician's Orders**, **History and Physical**, and **Nursing Admission** reports.

1. As you read these records, list the data that are consistent with bronchiolitis.

2. What do these observations indicate as far as Carrie's health status is concerned? In other words, how do you interpret the seriousness of her illness?

3. Refer to the Physician's Orders. What is the rationale for the orders for IV fluid, medications, oxygen, pulse oximety, and lab work?

4. Carrie had nasal washing done while she was in the ED. If you were performing the nasal washing procedure, would you anticipate restraining Carrie? If so, how? Would you have Carrie's mother help? What factors would you consider to help you to decide what to do? (*Hint:* Check Carrie's physical status and behavior while in the ED.)

5. Explain the type of isolation being used. (*Hint:* To find this, check the Physician's Orders in Carrie's chart.)

6. What other infection-control precautions need to be implemented?

 • Click on **Return to Nurses' Station** and then on Room **303** at the bottom of the screen.
 • Click on **Patient Care**.
 • Click on **Nurse-Client Interactions**.
 • Select and view the video titled **0730: Patient Assessment**. (*Note:* If this video is not available, check the virtual clock to see whether enough time has elapsed. The video cannot be viewed before its specified time.)

7. View the video clip. What is right or wrong with this picture?

Exercise 3

 CD-ROM Activity

45 minutes

- Sign in to work at Pacific View Regional Hospital on the Pediatrics Floor for Period of Care 1. (*Note:* If you are already in the virtual hospital from a previous exercise, click on **Leave the Floor** and then **Restart the Program** to get to the sign-in window.)
- From the Patient List, select Carrie Richards.
- Click on **Go to Nurses' Station**.
- Click on **303** to go to Carrie's room.
- Inside the room, click on **Check Armband** and then on **Take Vital Signs**. Note Carrie's vital signs for documentation.
- Next, click on **Patient Care** and do a head-to-toe assessment by clicking on the various body areas and subcategories.

1. Based on your assessment, list any observations that reflect Carrie's oxygenation status.

2. Carrie is of African-American descent. What is the best way to assess color in a dark-skinned person?

→ • Click on **EPR** and then on **Login**.

• Specify **303** in the Patient box.

• Begin charting the finding from your assessment of Carrie by selecting **Vital Signs** in the Category box. Use the blue backward and forward arrows as needed to document these data in the appropriate time column.

• Continue to chart your observations in the respiratory and cardiovascular areas.

3. If you missed anything, go back to Carrie's room and reassess her. Because the EPR format is generic, you may not have data for all areas listed. You do, though, need to make sure you are recognizing significant assessment data. Review data trends since admission. What is your assessment of Carrie's status? Why is continued monitoring necessary?

→ • Click **Exit EPR** to return to Carrie's room.

• Click on **Patient Care**.

• Based on your previous findings and your answer to question 3, perform a focused assessment of Carrie.

• Click on **Leave the Floor**.

• Click on **Look at Your Preceptor's Evaluations**.

• Click on **Examination Report**.

• Review the report. You may print the Examination Report if you wish.

4. How did you do with your focused assessment? Do you note any gaps? Were you efficient and systemic? Is there any area for improvement in your performance?

→ • Click on **Return to Evaluations**.

• Click on **Return to Menu** and **Restart the Program**.

• Sign in to work at Pacific View Regional Hospital on the Pediatric Floor for Period of Care 1.

• From the Patient List, select Carrie Richards.

• Click on **Go to Nurses' Station**.

• Click on **EPR** and then on **Login**.

• Select Carrie's EPR (**303**) and document your latest assessment findings.

5. Is Carrie's condition improving or deteriorating?

6. Consider the possibility of Carrie's condition deteriorating. What changes might you anticipate that would indicate worsening of her health status?

7. How is Carrie receiving oxygen?

8. Sometimes oxygen is delivered in a mist tent. What are the nursing responsibilities for care of an infant in a mist tent? Are there any advantages to using a mist tent rather than a nasal cannula?

9. How is Carrie's O_2 status being monitored? What should the nurse be looking for?

10. Documentation is important. What information is necessary for documenting observations associated with Carrie's O_2 saturation levels?

11. Oxygenation assessment is ongoing. In older children and adults, the nurse can easily assess respiratory status in response to play or other activity. How can this ongoing assessment be carried out in an infant?

Exercise 4

Clinical Preparation: Writing Activity

30 minutes

1. You have completed an oxygenation assessment. Write the priority nursing diagnosis for Carrie at this time. (*Hint:* You may find it useful to check distinguishing characteristics for the various oxygenation nursing diagnoses in a nursing diagnosis book. It is important to select an appropriate nursing diagnosis.)

2. Write goals with outcomes for your priority nursing diagnosis.

3. Develop nursing interventions for this nursing diagnosis. Make sure you include time frames and amounts where appropriate.

4. Evaluate your goals. Create an evaluation statement that reflects achievement of goals. (*Hint:* Specific outcomes need to be included here.)

5. Create an evaluation statement that reflects goals that are not met.

Congratulations! You have completed a comprehensive review of bronchiolitis and several aspects of nursing care. Proceed to Lesson 15 to learn about addressing other specific challenges in the care of an infant with a respiratory illness.

Nursing Care Issues Associated with Bronchiolitis

✐ **Reading Assignment:** Medicating Infants and Children
(Chapter 38, pages 970-976 and 983-986)
The Child with a Fluid and Electrolyte Alteration
(Chapter 42, pages 1079-1089)

Patient: Carrie Richards, Room 303

Goal: Demonstrate an understanding of other problems and care issues associated with bronchiolitis.

Objectives:

- Discuss the reasons why infants are at risk for hydration problems.
- Explain the risk for dehydration in infants with respiratory problems.
- Discuss nursing care for managing hydration concerns, including IV therapy.
- Practice oral medication administration in infants.
- Identify and discuss areas for independent teaching in the care of infants.
- Discuss discharge teaching responsibilities for the client with bronchiolitis.

In this lesson, you will explore hydration as an area of concern in infants with respiratory problems. You will also explore oral medication administration and practice it in a virtual sense. You will consider the role of the nurse related to a variety of teaching areas: the illness, oral administration of medications, and growth and development. You will need to recall and use the principles of good communication and family teaching as you continue to work with Carrie Richards.

Exercise 1

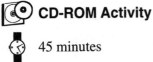 **CD-ROM Activity**

45 minutes

1. List the characteristics of infants that put them at greater risk for hydration problems. Include and underline those that particularly relate to dehydration as a potential problem with respiratory illness.

2. List the areas you would want to assess in completing a hydration assessment.

→ • Sign in to work at Pacific View Regional Hospital on the Pediatrics Floor for Period of Care 1. (*Note:* If you are already in the virtual hospital from a previous exercise, click on **Leave the Floor** and then **Restart the Program** to get to the sign-in window.)

• From the Patient List, select Carrie Richards.

• Click on **Get Report** and then on **Go to Nurses' Station**.

• Click on **303** at the bottom of your screen.

• Click on **Patient Care** and complete a focused assessment of Carrie. (*Remember:* A focused assessment is one that reflects the priority health concern as well as those concerns for which the patient is at risk.)

• Once your assessment is complete, click on **EPR** and then on **Login**.

• Specifiy Carrie's room number (**303**) and choose categories as needed to record the data from your focused assessment. (*Hint:* If you need help entering data in the EPR, refer to pages 15-16 in the **Getting Started** section of this workbook.)

• When you have finished documenting your assessments, click on **Exit EPR**.

• Now, to see how you did, click on **Leave the Floor**.

• From the Floor Menu, select **Look at Your Preceptor's Evaluations**.

• Now click on **Examination Report** and review the feedback.

3. Reflect on your performance with this assessment. Did you assess respiratory status along with hydration parameters? Remember that one affects the other.

4. What important hydration assessment parameters can you use with Carrie that would not be available with an older child?

5. What is the most reliable information you can use to assess an infant's hydration over time? Why?

Now let's jump ahead in virtual time to practice your focused assessment again.

➤ • Click on **Return to Evaluations**, then on **Return to Menu**, and then on **Restart the Program**.
  • Sign in to work with Carrie Richards for Period of Care 2.
  • Click on **Go to Nurses' Station** and then on **303** to go to Carrie's room.
  • Complete a focused assessment and then chart your findings on the appropriate flow sheets in the EPR. (*Hint:* If you need help entering data in the EPR, refer to pages 15-16 in the **Getting Started** section of this workbook.)
  • When you have finished documenting your assessments, click on **Exit EPR**.
  • Now, to see how you did, click on **Leave the Floor**.
  • From the Floor Menu, select **Look at Your Preceptor's Evaluations**.
  • Now click on **Examination Report** and review the feedback.

6. Reflect on how you are doing with your focused assessment. Consider completeness, comfort, efficiency and skill. Are you feeling more confident about your thoroughness?

Now practice your focused assessment once more, this time in Period of Care 3.

➤ • Once again, click on **Return to Evaluations**, then on **Return to Menu**, and then on **Restart the Program**.
  • Sign in to work with Carrie Richards for Period of Care 3.
  • Click on **Go to Nurses' Station** and then on **303** to go to Carrie's room.
  • Complete a focused assessment and then chart your findings on the appropriate flow sheets in the EPR. (*Hint:* If you need help entering data in the EPR, refer to pages 15-16 in the **Getting Started** section of this workbook.)
  • When you have finished documenting your assessments, click on **Exit EPR**.
  • Now, to see how you did, click on **Leave the Floor**.
  • From the Floor Menu, select **Look at Your Preceptor's Evaluations**.
  • Now click on **Examination Report** and review the feedback.

7. Once more, reflect on how you are doing with your focused assessment. What improvements have you made? What have you learned? Is there still room for more improvement?

8. Discuss the nursing responsibilities associated with IV fluid administration in infants. (*Hint:* Remember that IV fluid is treated as a medication administration.)

9. What should the nurse be looking for when assessing an IV site?

10. You find that infusion pumps are in very short supply. You know that Carrie, because of her age, needs a pump and she will get the next available one. In the meantime, you must anticipate using IV tubing that has a burette. What is the rationale for use of this type of tubing?

➔ • Click on **Chart** and then on **303**.
   • Click on **Nursing Admissions**.

11. Calculate Carrie's daily fluid maintenance needs. (*Hint:* You will need to find Carrie's weight in the Nursing Admissions form to make this calculation.)

12. What would you tell Carrie's Mom about adequate hydration? How she will know whether her baby is getting enough fluids?

→ • Now click on **Physician's Orders**. Find the most recent order for IV fluids for Carrie.

13. Carrie is receiving an IV infusion with potassium added. Explain what she is receiving. Discuss the nurse's responsibilities related to potassium administration to an infant.

14. Consider what aspects of care (with regard to managing the IV) you may delegate to Carrie's mother. What could you ask her to do while still maintaining safe care and fulfilling your legal responsibility?

15. Explain what is meant by oral rehydration therapy.

Exercise 2

 CD-ROM Activity

30 minutes

- Sign in to work at Pacific View Regional Hospital on the Pediatrics Floor for Period of Care 3. (*Note:* If you are already in the virtual hospital from a previous exercise, click on **Leave the Floor** and then **Restart the Program** to get to the sign-in window.)
- From the Patient List, select Carrie Richards.
- Click on **Go to Nurses' Station**.
- Click on **303** to go to Carrie's room.
- Click on **Take Vital Signs**.
- Click on **Clinical Alerts** and review the report.

1. Can Carrie have Tylenol? If so, for what reason will you be giving it?

2. What do you want to assess/check before you prepare the medication? (*Hint:* Consider the specific need for this medication, as well as the nursing responsibilities before administering any medication.)

→ • Click on **MAR** and find the order for this medication.

3. Is the ordered dose of this medication appropriate for Carrie? If not, why not?

4. Assume that Carrie had an order for an antibiotic that read "40 mg/kg/day PO in divided doses every 8 hours." How much would you give for each dose?

5. What are the appropriate methods for administering oral medications to an infant?

- Click on **Return to Room 303**.
- Click on **Medication Room**.
- Click on **Unit Dosage**.
- Click on drawer **303**.
- Click on **Acetaminophen**.
- Click on **Put Medication on Tray**.
- Click on **Close Drawer**.
- Click on **View Medication Room**.
- Click on **Preparation**.
- Click on **Prepare** and follow the Preparation Wizard's prompts to complete preparation of Carrie's acetaminophen dose.
- Click on **Return to Medication Room**.
- Click on **303** to return to Carrie's room.
- Click on **Check Armband**.
- Click on **Check Allergies**.
- Click on **Patient Care**.
- Click on **Medication Administration**.
- Find **Acetaminophen** listed on the left side of your screen. To its right, click on the down arrow next to **Select** and choose **Administer**.
- Follow the Administration Wizard's prompts to administer the medication. Indicate **Yes** to document the injection in the MAR.
- Click on **Leave the Floor**.
- Click on **Look at Your Preceptor's Evaluation**.
- Click on **Medication Scorecard**. How did you do?

6. Did you get check marks indicating that you completed the medication administration procedure satisfactorily? What, if anything, did you forget? What, if anything, would you do differently?

You have just been walked through the medication preparation and administration procedure. Now try it on your own. To do so, you have two options:

- Click on **MAR** and see whether Carrie has any other medications due at this time. If she does, you can stay in this period of care and proceed with the preparation and administration.
- If you prefer to practice preparing and giving Carrie the same acetaminophen dose you just completed, click on **Leave the Floor** and then **Restart the Program**. Sign in again to work with Carrie for Period of Care 3 and proceed from there.

Regardless of which option you choose, remember to follow the Five Rights! After you have finished administering the medication, be sure to see how you did by checking your Medication Scorecard:

- Click on **Leave the Floor** and then on **Look at Your Preceptor's Evaluations**.
- Click on **Medication Scorecard** and review your evaluation.

Now let's jump backward in virtual time to visit Carrie earlier in the day.

- First, click on **Return to Evaluations**, then on **Return to Menu**, and then on **Restart the Program**.
- Sign in to work with Carrie Richards again, this time for Period of Care 2.
- Click on **Go to Nurses' Station** and then on **303** to go to Carrie's room.
- Click on **Patient Care** and then on **Nurse-Client Interactions**.
- Select and view the video titled **1115: Nutritional Assessment**.

7. Share your thoughts on your assessment of the nurse's teaching. Consider the teaching-learning principles that are depicted.

8. Carrie's mother needs to know how to give her infant medication at home. How will you determine whether she is skillful and comfortable enough giving her baby medication?

9. How would you respond to the following concern: "The nurse is supposed to give the medication, so how can the nurse allow a parent to administer medication?" (*Hint:* To answer this, you need to think through the nurse's legal responsibilities.)

Exercise 3

 Clinical Preparation: Writing Activity

15 minutes

1. What are the topics you will want to include in discharge instructions after hospitalization with bronchiolitis?

2. These topics represent the content that needs to be taught. What about methods you will use? What will you do to ensure teaching is understood?

3. Providing anticipatory guidance is very important. Carrie is 3½ months old. Identify some changes her mother should anticipate in the next few weeks.

4. The only vaccine Carrie has received is for hepatitis B. What teaching does Carrie's mother need with regard to immunizations?

Great job on completing this lesson! The content to which you have been exposed has helped you think about pediatric situations in the hospital setting.

Caring for an Infant Failing to Thrive

👓 **Reading Assignment:** Read about **infant nutrition** (Chapter 5, pages 89-93) and **failure to thrive** (Chapter 53, pages 1550 and 1555-1558).

Patient: Carrie Richards, Room 303

Goal: Demonstrate an understanding of management of failure to thrive and family-centered care.

Objectives:

- Discuss nutritional needs of the infant.
- Define failure to thrive (FTT).
- Consider patterns of growth that may indicate FTT.
- Determine areas of assessment when FTT is suspected.
- Discuss relationship of parenting skills to FTT.
- Develop specific interventions for caring for an infant with FTT.

As you complete this lesson, you will be exploring the complexities of failure to thrive, including the factors of parent-infant interaction and parenting skills. You will consider the role of the nurse in assessment, support, and teaching when providing care.

Exercise 1

✎ **Clinical Preparation: Writing Activity**

🕐 15 minutes

1. Why is adequate nutrition so important in infancy?

2. What should Carrie's nutritional intake be like at 3½ months of age?

3. Differentiate between organic and nonorganic failure to thrive.

4. The following is a lengthy list of assessment data. Some data are physiologic, and some are psychosocial. Read the list and place an X next to all that should be assessed when there is a concern about failure to thrive.

_____ a. Weight less than 5th percentile

_____ b. Sudden deceleration in growth

_____ c. Delay in reaching milestones

_____ d. Decreased muscle mass

_____ e. Muscle hypotonia

_____ f. Abdominal distention

_____ g. General weakness

_____ h. Cachexia

_____ i. Avoidance of eye contact or touch

_____ j. Intense watchfulness

_____ k. Sleep disturbance

_____ l. Lack of age-appropriate stranger anxiety

_____ m. Lack of preference for parents

_____ n. Repetitive self-stimulating behavior

Exercise 2

 CD-ROM Activity

15 minutes

- Sign in to work at Pacific View Regional Hospital on the Pediatrics Floor for Period of Care 2. (*Note:* If you are already in the virtual hospital from a previous exercise, click on **Leave the Floor** and then **Restart the Program** to get to the sign-in window.)
- From the Patient List, select Carrie Richards.
- Click on **Go to Nurses' Station**.
- Click on **Chart** and then on **303**.
- Click on **Nursing Admission**.

1. Review Carrie's chart for growth information. Plot her length and weight on the growth chart found on page 1614 in your text. In what percentile does Carrie fall? Does this assessment help you to see where there is a problem? Can you now visualize what Carrie looks like?

2. If you knew Carrie's birth weight, how would you use the data? What is the rule of thumb for expected weight gain in an infant?

- Now click on **Consultations**.
- Review the Dietary/Nutrition Consult.

3. Find Carrie's birth weight. Based on this information, what concerns do you have about her rate of growth?

4. You have considered the recommended diet for a 3½-month old in question 2 of Exercise 1 in this lesson. How does this compare with Carrie's actual diet? Evaluate the adequacy of Carrie's diet and consider her mother's rationales for these choices. Is there anything else you want to know/assess?

5. Based on your review of the Dietary/Nutrition Consult, what do you think is the problem in regard to Carrie's feedings? What additional dietary recommendations are planned for Carrie?

6. As you talk with Carrie's mother, you learn that income is a problem. When discussing feeding, what should you incorporate in your teaching?

7. How will you implement teaching about formula preparation for Carrie's mother?

Exercise 3

 CD-ROM Activity

35 minutes

- Sign in to work at Pacific View Regional Hospital on the Pediatrics Floor for Period of Care 1. (*Note:* If you are already in the virtual hospital from a previous exercise, click on **Leave the Floor** and then **Restart the Program** to get to the sign-in window.)
- From the Patient List, select Carrie Richards.
- Click on **Go to Nurses' Station**.
- Click on **Chart** and then on **303**.
- Review the **History and Physical**.

1. In the previous exercise, you learned about the following assessment data for failure to thrive. Which of these specifically apply to Carrie? Based on your review of her chart, place an X next to any data that are known in Carrie's case.

_____ a. Weight less than 5th percentile

_____ b. Sudden deceleration in growth

_____ c. Delay in reaching milestones

_____ d. Decreased muscle mass

_____ e. Muscle hypotonia

_____ f. Abdominal distention

_____ g. General weakness

_____ h. Cachexia

_____ i. Avoidance of eye contact or touch

_____ j. Intense watchfulness

_____ k. Sleep disturbance

_____ l. Lack of age-appropriate stranger anxiety

_____ m. Lack of preference for parents

_____ n. Repetitive self-stimulating behaviors

- Select and view the video titled **0755: Intervention—Weight**. (*Note:* If this video is not available, check the virtual clock to see whether enough time has elapsed. The video cannot be viewed before its specified time.)

2. How should the nurse weigh Carrie? Why has she elected to obtain the weight before feeding? After all, Carrie has been fussy and seems to want to be fed.

 • Now select and view the video titled **0800: Assessment—Fact Finding**.

3. What do you think the nurse is planning to assess as she observes the mother feeding Carrie?

4. Why is it essential to know that Carrie's mother is able to respond to her infant's cues and correctly interpret them?

5. Are there other areas you would like to explore in this situation? If so, what are they?

Exercise 4

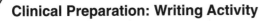 **Clinical Preparation: Writing Activity**

15 minutes

Review the Nursing Care Plan on pages 1556-1557 in your text. This care plan addresses growth in the infant as well as knowledge deficit in the parent. Pay particular attention to the areas of ongoing assessment and monitoring.

1. Based on what you have learned in previous exercises, what other nursing diagnosis might be appropriate for Carrie's mother? (*Hint:* Consider the lack of resources available to her.)

2. Create a short-term goal for Carrie's mother with specific outcome criteria.

3. Develop nursing interventions to help achieve the criteria you identified in question 2.

4. Write an evaluative statement that reflects meeting the goal you created in question 2.

5. Discuss the nature of interdisciplinary collaboration in this situation. Who are the players, and what might the outcomes be in anticipation of discharge?

Exercise 5

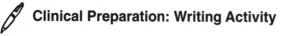 **Clinical Preparation: Writing Activity**

15 minutes

1. What if you noticed that Carrie's mother always had the TV on while feeding Carrie and seemed to pay more attention to the TV than to Carrie? How would you intervene?

2. Refer to page 1547 in your text. The definition of child abuse refers to emotional abuse, physical abuse, and neglect. Is there abuse in this situation? Is there risk for abuse? Share your reasons for thinking the way you do.

3. Envision yourself working with Carrie's mother. How do you feel toward her? What do you think it would be like to carry out the teaching plans articulated? (*Hint:* Think about what the term "Rescue Fantasy" means to you.)

Caring for a Young Child with Meningitis

👓 **Reading Assignment:** Read about **meningitis** (Chapter 52, pages 1522-1525) and **lumbar puncture** (Chapter 51, pages 1490-1491).

Patient: Stephanie Brown, Room 304

Goal: Demonstrate an understanding of nursing care for a child with meningitis.

Objectives:

- Describe the pathophysiology of meningitis.
- Discuss risk factors for meningitis.
- List assessment data indicative of meningitis.
- Explain rationale for treatment of meningitis.
- Develop a care plan for a child with meningitis.
- Discuss strategies for supporting a parent and child through diagnosis and treatment.

In this lesson, you will learn about the problem of meningitis in a child and nursing care. You will focus on a variety of challenges associated with this problem. You may need to review the concepts of growth and development of a young child, as well as teaching-learning principles.

Exercise 1

💿 **CD-ROM Activity**

⌚ 45 minutes

 1. Review the pathophysiology information on page 1523 of your text. Explain the pathophysiology of meningitis in terms that a parent could understand.

→ • Sign in to work at Pacific View Regional Hospital on the Pediatrics Floor for Period of Care 1. (*Note:* If you are already in the virtual hospital from a previous exercise, click on **Leave the Floor** and then **Restart the Program** to get to the sign-in window.)

• From the Patient List, select Stephanie Brown.

• Click on **Get Report**.

• Click on **Go to Nurses' Station**.

• Click on **Chart** and then on **304** for Stephanie Brown's record.

• Review the following sections of the chart: **Physician's Notes**, **Emergency Department**, **History and Physical**, and **Nursing Admission**.

2. Given the information you have learned about Stephanie and her family, reflect on your response to question 1. Would you change anything? If your answer is yes, what would you change and how would you present the information? If the answer is no, identify the strengths reflected in your teaching about the diagnosis. Make sure your response reflects some of the information you have learned that affects teaching in this situation. Incorporate other teaching-learning principles as they apply.

3. What in Stephanie's situation increases her risk for developing meningitis?

4. What assessment data on admissions did Stephanie exhibit that would indicate a diagnosis of meningitis?

5. What additional assessments would you make?

6. If Stephanie had this diagnosis, what other assessments could you perform?

7. In addition to nuchal rigidity, positive responses to two other signs were elicited from

   Stephanie that are indicative of meningitis. They are _____ and

   _____ signs.

8. Explain how each of the signs listed below are tested. Then briefly describe the response each sign would elicit in a child with meningitis.

Sign	To Test for Sign	Response in Meningitis
Nuchal rigidity		
Kernig's sign		
Brudzinski's sign		

➤ • Still in Stephanie's chart, click on **Physician's Orders** and review.
   • Then click on **Diagnostic Reports** and review.

9. What test is diagnostic for meningitis? What data are consistent with a diagnosis of meningitis?

10. Discuss the types of meningitis most commonly seen in childhood. Incorporate etiologic factors in your answer.

11. Which type of meningitis is associated with droplet transmission and increased risk for infection as exposure to contacts expands?

12. Match each of the following physician's orders with its rationale.

Physician's Order	**Rationale**
_____ Pulse oximetry q4h	a. Baseline—aminoglycosides can cause ototoxicity
_____ Neuro checks q4h	b. Gravity reduces intracranial pressure
_____ Blood culture for fever above 101°	c. Used to maintain therapeutic blood level
_____ Audiogram	d. Monitoring of neurologic status
_____ Keep HOB elevated 45 degrees	e. Disease can be transmitted via droplets
_____ Respiratory isolation	f. Assessment for other causative agents
_____ Vancomycin levels	g. Ongoing monitoring of O_2 status

Exercise 2

 CD-ROM Activity

60 minutes

- Sign in to work at Pacific View Regional Hospital on the Pediatrics Floor for Period of Care 1. (*Note:* If you are already in the virtual hospital from a previous exercise, click on **Leave the Floor** and then **Restart the Program** to get to the sign-in window.)
- From the Patient List, select Stephanie Brown.
- Click on **Go to Nurses' Station** and then on **304** to visit Stephanie.
- Inside her room, click on **Patient Care**.
- Complete a focused assessment of Stephanie's neurologic status.
- When you finish your assessment, click on **Leave the Floor**.
- From the Floor Menu, select **Look at Your Preceptor's Evaluations**.
- Next, click on **Examination Report** and review the feedback.

1. Reflect on your assessment skills. Did you miss any areas?

➡ - To return to the Pediatrics Floor, click on **Return to Evaluations** and then on **Return to Menu**.
- From the Floor Menu, click on **Restart the Program**.
- Sign in to work with Stephanie Brown for Period of Care 2.
- Click on **Go to Nurses' Station**.
- Click on Room **304**.
- Click on **Patient Care**.
- Click on **Nurse-Client Interactions**.
- Select and view the video titled **1120: Preventing Spread of Disease**. (*Note:* If this video is not available, check the virtual clock to see whether enough time has elapsed. The video cannot be viewed before its specified time.)

2. CDC guidelines require standard precautions for all types of meningitis, as well as droplet precautions for certain types. What else needs to be included to effectively implement droplet precautions?

3. The above guidelines are implemented right away and kept in place until 24 hours after antibiotics have been started. Antibiotics are always administered before the cultures come back. Why?

4. What kind of isolation was the nurse in the video using? Was this correct and consistent with the physician's orders?

5. Suppose that you see Stephanie's mother not wearing a mask. When you ask her about this, she says she doesn't need to do anything special because she never leaves Stephanie's room. How would you respond?

• Now select and view the video titled **1145: Teaching—Disease Sequelae**.

6. Discuss the most common potential sequelae associated with meningitis. Incorporate the mechanism of injury in your answer.

7. Is Stephanie on any treatment or medication that may contribute to permanent injury?

 • Click on **Chart** and then on **304**.
 • Click on **Physician's Orders**.

8. Review Stephanie's IV orders. Calculate the total volume for 24 hours.

 • Click on **Return to Room 304**.
 • Next, click on **Leave the Floor** and then on **Restart the Program**.
 • Sign in to work with Stephanie Brown again, this time for Period of Care 3.
 • Click on **Go to Nurses' Station**.
 • Click on Room **304**.
 • Click on **Patient Care**.
 • Click on **Nurse-Client Interactions**.
 • Select and view the video titled **1510: Nurse-Patient Communication**. (*Note:* If this video is not available, check the virtual clock to see whether enough time has elapsed. The video cannot be viewed before its specified time.)

9. What is the nurse's assessment and decision?

10. The nurse explains to Stephanie that she is going to apply a local anesthetic. What is a more age-appropriate way of saying this?

11. What is the anesthetic being used? How is it used in order to be most effective?

12. Notice the nurse's interaction with Stephanie and her mother. Why is Stephanie, who is only 3 years old, included in the explanation?

13. At Stephanie's age, how might she perceive her hospital experience? How might she percieve the nurse?

14. Notice Stephanie's mother's behavior. How might that affect Stephanie's perceptions?

15. From a developmental perspective, what are major fears of children in Stephanie's age group? What behaviors might the child display?

16. What strategies can you employ to promote a more positive experience for Stephanie?

Exercise 3

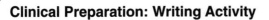

Clinical Preparation: Writing Activity

15 minutes

1. Explain the issue of prophylaxis for anyone who has had close contact with a patient who has meningitis.

2. Think about how you might respond to any questions that Stephanie's daycare provider might have. What issues should be discussed?

3. Let's assume that Stephanie has had a relapse and is now doing worse. Other family members have been taking turns staying with her. She still has an IV and is very restless and irritable. Even the family members are getting irritable, and they express concern about all the babies on the unit that have to be fed and cared for. They worry about Stephanie receiving the care she needs. How will you help them?

Caring for a Young Child with Cerebral Palsy

Reading Assignment: Read about **cerebral palsy** (Chapter 52, pages 1508-1512) and **DDST-II** (Chapter 4, pages 62-63). Review **growth and development** of the young child (Chapter 6, pages 103-127).

Patient: Stephanie Brown, Room 304

Goal: Demonstrate an understanding of caring for a child with cerebral palsy.

Objectives:

- Describe the behaviors and problems associated with the most common types of cerebral palsy (CP).
- Discuss a range of etiologic factors associated with cerebral palsy.
- Explain the importance of early diagnosis and treament to the child's optimal level of function.
- Discuss the nursing care needs of a child with cerebral palsy.

Completing this lesson will help you gain an appreciation of the challenges associated with caring for a child who has cerebral palsy—both for parents and for the nurse. You will also explore the issue of encountering cerebral palsy as a condition that coexists with other health problems, the latter being the reason for hospitalization or other health care encounter. You will be working with Stephanie Brown in Room 304.

Exercise 1

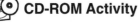 **CD-ROM Activity**

30 minutes

- Sign in to work at Pacific View Regional Hospital on the Pediatrics Floor for Period of Care 1. (*Note:* If you are already in the virtual hospital from a previous exercise, click on **Leave the Floor** and then **Restart the Program** to get to the sign-in window.)
- From the Patient List, select Stephanie Brown.
- Click on **Get Report**.
- Click on **Go to Nurses' Station**.

1. You may have a very general understanding of cerebral palsy. Perhaps you think you have encountered kids with this condition in your personal and professional life and remember thinking that these children look challenging to care for. What is cerebral palsy?

2. What types of fine and gross motor functions may be affected by cerebral palsy?

→ • Click on **304** to go to Stephanie's room.
   • Click on **Patient Care** and perform a focused assessment.

3. Based on your assessment of Stephanie, list any behavioral responses she demonstrates that are associated with CP.

→ • Click on Chart and then on **304**.
   • Click on the **History and Physical** tab.

4. Review Stephanie's history. What might be an etiologic factor in Stephanie's situation?

5. Early recognition and treatment are important to fostering achievement of optimal development. Why is cerebral palsy often not diagnosed until about 2 years of age?

→ • Click on **Return to Room 304**.
   • Click on **Patient Care**.
   • Click on **Nurse-Client Interactions**.
   • Select and view the video titled **0750: Caring for the Child with CP**. (*Note:* If this video is not available, check the virtual clock to see whether enough time has elapsed. The video cannot be viewed before its specified time.)

6. What is the nurse doing as she listens to Stephanie's mother explain problems Stephanie has that are associated with cerebral palsy.

7. Should the nurse be supportive of Stephanie's mother implementing the treatments and strategies she uses at home? Why or why not?

8. What problem is Stephanie at risk for during her hospitalization? (*Hint:* You will need to consider Stephanie's developmental age.)

→ • Click on **Chart** and then on **304**.
   • Click on **Nursing Admission** and review for data about Stephanie's development.

9. Hospitalization can still be a time of growth. Explore which developmental tasks Stephanie has achieved and which she has not. Comment on her development.

10. This is a good opportunity to explore Stephanie's development further. Assume Stephanie has recently turned 3 years of age. Using the DDST-II score sheet found on pages 1619-1621 of your text, determine one skill that Stephanie should have completed, one that she is working on, and one that she is not yet ready for. Do this in one of the four skill areas. (*Hint:* You may want to review how to use the DDST-II first.)

Exercise 2

 CD-ROM Activity

30 minutes

- Sign in to work at Pacific View Regional Hospital on the Pediatrics Floor for Period of Care 3. (*Note:* If you are already in the virtual hospital from a previous exercise, click on **Leave the Floor** and then **Restart the Program** to get to the sign-in window.)
- From the Patient List, select Stephanie Brown.
- Click on **Get Report**.
- Click on **Go to Nurses' Station**.
- Click on **Chart** and then on **304**.
- Review Stephanie's records, in particular her **History and Physical**.

1. What type of cerebral palsy does Stephanie have? What are the signs that she manifests?

2. Match each type of cerebral palsy with its description.

Type	Description
_____ Spastic	a. Rigid flexor and extensor muscles; tremors
_____ Dyskinetic/athetoid	b. Increased deep tendon reflexes, hypertonia, flexion, and scissors gait
_____ Ataxic	c. Slow, writhing uncontrolled and involuntary movements
_____ Rigid	d. Loss of coordination, equilibrium, and kinesthetic sense

3. Cerebral palsy can have an impact on many aspects of the child's life. A number of problems can be associated with the behaviors the child manifests. What are some of these? Make sure that at least one is a psychosocial concern.

4. What if Stephanie's mother expresses guilt over her condition, saying she knows now that she did some things that may have contributed to the condition? How would you respond? (*Hint:* You may want to review your response to question 4 in Exercise 1 of this lesson.)

 5. In general, what is the etiology of cerebral palsy? For specific factors, refer to the list in the box on page 1509 in your textbook. What do these factors have in common?

6. Assume that Stephanie's mother asks you whether you see any signs of mental retardation in her daughter. She is worried that this will develop as Stephanie's disease progresses. What can you tell her? How will you reassure her?

→ • Click on **Return to Nurses' Station**.
  • Click on Room **304**.
  • Click on **Patient Care** and then on **Nurse-Client Interactions**.
  • Select and view the video titled **1530: Preventive Measures**. (*Note:* If this video is not available, check the virtual clock to see whether enough time has elapsed. The video cannot be viewed before its specified time.)

7. Why does Stephanie require heel cord stretching?

8. What other preventive measures have been integrated into Stephanie's regimen to prevent complications associated with cerebral palsy?

9. What is the nursing role with regard to supporting these endeavors?

10. Explain why nutrition is so important for the child who has cerebral palsy.

11. Nurses are frequently asked for advice. Stephanie's mother sends her daughter to a preschool program but wonders whether it is the best school for her. What advice can you give her?

Exercise 3

Clinical Preparation: Writing Activity

30 minutes

1. When children are hospitalized for an acute illness, you may find that the child also has some other disability or chronic illness that could have an effect on the hospitalization or your care. Think about how you would provide care in such a situation. How do you get information? Who is in charge? Do you involve parents in the same ways you usually do? How do you feel about people with disabilities? Reflect and respond.

2. Develop a plan to teach Stephanie's mother to promote self-esteem as Stephanie progresses through the stage of initiative versus guilt. First, write one or more goals.

3. Now develop nursing interventions designed to meet the goal(s) you wrote in question 2. (*Hint:* See the box on page 134 of your textbook. Some of these ideas can be adapted.)

4. Does your community have a Children with Special Care Needs/Early Intervention Program? What do you think the program is about?

5. Visit *www.ucp.org* and then respond to the following questions:

   a. What did you like or not like about the site?

b. To whom is this site geared?

c. What did you learn that was new information?

d. Would you recommend this site to parents of a child with cerebral palsy? Why or why not?

Caring for a School-Age Child with Diabetes Mellitus

————————————————————————————

Reading Assignment: Read about **diabetes mellitus** (Chapter 51, pages 1466-1485).

Patient: George Gonzalez, Room 301

Goal: Demonstrate an understanding of managing diabetes mellitus in a child.

Objectives:

- Discuss the pathophysiology of diabetes mellitus.
- Compare and contrast type 1 and type 2 diabetes.
- Explain the role of insulin in the metabolism of foods.
- Discuss management and nursing responsibilities for insulin therapy, diet, exercise, and blood glucose monitoring.
- Contrast causes, signs, and management of hypoglycemia and hyperglycemia.
- Explain the pathophysiology of diabetic ketoacidosis (DKA) and discuss its management and nursing care.
- Discuss the impact of growth and development on diabetes.

Most likely, you have had instruction in diabetes and have a basic understanding of the disease and its problems. In this lesson, you will work with 11-year-old George Gonzales in Room 301. You will learn more about diabetes by considering problems and nursing care based on the current status of George's illness. In doing so, you will need to apply principles of growth and development. Although teaching may be touched on, the teaching-learning process as it relates to this situation will be discussed in more depth in the following lesson. You may need to review concepts of growth and development.

Exercise 1

 CD-ROM Activity

55 minutes

- Sign in to work at Pacific View Regional Hospital on the Pediatrics Floor for Period of Care 1. (*Note:* If you are already in the virtual hospital from a previous exercise, click on **Leave the Floor** and then **Restart the Program** to get to the sign-in window.)
- From the Patient List, select George Gonzalez.
- Click on **Go to Nurses' Station**.

- Click on **Chart** and then on **301** for George Gonzalez's record.
- Click on **Emergency Department** and review this record.

1. George has been admitted with a diagnosis of diabetic ketoacidosis (DKA). What does this mean?

2. What makes George at particular risk for developing diabetes?

3. Match the following to show your understanding of the differences between type 1 and type 2 diabetes.

Characteristic	**Type**
_____ Most common childhood endocrine disease	a. Type 1 diabetes
_____ Results from autoimmune process disorder	b. Type 2 diabetes
_____ Cells are unable to use insulin	
_____ Genetic predisposition is a factor	
_____ Pancreas is unable to produce insulin	
_____ Obesity commonly coexists	

4. What symptoms was George likely to be having at the onset of his illness 4 years ago? (*Hint:* Be sure to consider growth and development in your discussion.)

5. What are the signs of diabetic ketoacidosis (DKA)?

6. What was George's condition like when he was admitted? Was there a precipitating factor?

7. What will be the focus of care for the first portion of George's hospitalization for DKA?

8. What type of insulin is used and why? Identify any nursing concerns with the administration of insulin IV.

9. What are the signs of hyperglycemia?

10. What are the signs of hypoglycemia?

11. George is being treated for advanced hyperglycemia. What are the indications for treatment of hyperglycemia in the early stage? In the later stage?

12. For which of the following nursing diagnoses is there evidence in George's situation? Provide the data that lead you to this nursing diagnosis.

   a. Fluid volume deficit related to abnormal fluid losses through diuresis and emesis.
   b. Risk for injury from altered acid-base balance leading to ketone production and acidosis related to lack of insulin.
   c. Knowledge deficit related to unfamiliarity with home management during sick days.

13. What ongoing assessments need to be made?

14. What evidence is there that George's diabetes is out of control?

15. What is HBA1C? Explain its use as a diagnostic and teaching tool.

 • Click on **Return to Nurses' Station**.
   • Click on Room **301** at the bottom of the screen.
   • Click on **Patient Care**.
   • Click on **Nurse-Client Interactions**.
   • Select and view the video titled **0730: Supervision—Glucose Testing**.

16. What did the nurse do that facilitated George's honesty about his testing behavior and how he feels about it?

17. What is the nurse trying to accomplish when she asks George to do his own finger stick? (*Hint:* Consider developmental tasks of the school-age child.)

18. What is George's developmental stage? How might this affect his compliance with treatment plans?

→ • Select and view the video titled **0745: Self-Administering Insulin**. (*Note:* If this video is not available, check the virtual clock to see whether enough time has elapsed. The video cannot be viewed before its specified time.)

19. What does the nurse do that is positive as she observes George give his injection?

George needs insulin. Before going to the Medication Room, complete any necessary assessments.

→ • Click on **MAR** to check the order for insulin; then click on **Return to Room 301**.
  • Click on **Medication Room**.
  • Using the Five Rights, prepare the correct dose of insulin for George. When you have prepared the medication, return to George's room and administer it, again following the Five Rights. (*Hint:* Try to perform these steps on your own. If you need help, refer to pages 26-30 and 37-41 in the **Getting Started** section of this workbook.)
  • After administering the insulin, click on **Leave the Floor** and then on **Look at Your Preceptor's Evaluations**.
  • Next, click on **Medication Scorecard** and review the feedback.

20. Identify the things you need to do, if any, to satisfactorily complete the procedure.

- Click on **Return to Evaluations** and then on **Return to Menu**.
- Click on **Restart the Program.**
- Sign in to work with George Gonzalez for Period of Care 1.
- Click on **Go to Nurses' Station**.

21. Match each type of insulin with its corresponding characteristics.

Characteristic of Medication	Type of Insulin
_____ Onset of 30-60 minutes	a. Regular
_____ Onset of 2-4 hours	b. NPH
_____ Peak at 4-10 hours	
_____ Peak at 2-3 hours	
_____ Duration of 3-6 hours	
_____ Duration of 10-16 hours	

22. At what point during the day is George most at risk for a hypoglycemic reaction?

- Click on **Chart** and then on **301**.
- Click on **Physician's Orders**. Find the order for George's morning dose of insulin.

23. Using George's morning insulin order, describe the steps for drawing up two forms of insulin in one syringe.

24. Why is the short-acting insulin always drawn up first?

25. How should George be advised to rotate injection sites?

26. What are some possible barriers to compliance?

Let's jump ahead in virtual time to review and reinforce your insulin administration skills.

→ • Click on **Leave the Floor** and then on **Restart the Program**.
   • Sign in to work at Pacific View Regional Hospital on the Pediatrics Floor for Period of Care 2.
   • From the Patient List, select George Gonzalez.
   • Click on **Go to Nurses' Station**.
   • Once again, prepare and administer George's morning dose of insulin. Using the Five Rights, be sure to check the order, as well as George's blood glucose level. Perform the proper identification checks before giving the medication.
   • After administering the insulin, check your performance by reviewing the preceptor's Medication Scorecard.

27. Reflect on your performance. Consider the actual practice you may need in order to feel comfortable with this skill.

28. Off the top of your head, list the learning needs of a patient newly diagnosed with diabetes.

 29. Now refer to the list of learning needs on page 1473 in your textbook. How did you do with your list in question 28? Consider any needs you left off your list. Why do you think they were more difficult to remember?

30. Which of the above learning needs do George and his family currently have?

31. What anticipatory guidance can you offer George's mother with regard to how insulin needs change as George moves toward adolescence?

32. Discuss the relationship among insulin, food, and exercise. Explain it in terms that would be understandable by George and his family.

Let's jump ahead to visit George a little later in the day.

→ • To return to the Pediatrics Floor, click on **Return to Evaluations**, **Return to Menu**, and **Restart the Program**.

• Sign in to work with George Gonzalez, this time for Period of Care 2.

• Click on **Go to Nurses' Station**.

• Click on Room **301**.

• Click on **Patient Care**.

• Click on **Nurse-Client Interactions**.

• Select and view the video titled **1115: Teaching—Disease Process**. (*Note:* If this video is not available, check the virtual clock to see whether enough time has elapsed. The video cannot be viewed before its specified time.)

33. What are the sequelae of untreated or poorly managed diabetes? Explain why they occur.

Exercise 2

 Clinical Preparation: Writing Activity

15 minutes

1. You are a nurse in a physician's office. More and more treatment is occurring on an out-patient basis. Why do you think this is occurring? What are some approaches for responding to learning needs of children such as George Gonzalez?

2. Compare and contrast two or more websites designed for individuals with diabetes and their families. Write about the target group, ease of use, and appropriateness for suggesting to patients with diabetes and their families. You may do a search and select your own websites or choose from the following established sites:
   - *www.diabetes.org*
   - *www.idcdiabetes.org*
   - *www.jdrf.org*
   - *www.niddk.nih.gov*

3. Discuss how you could suggest involving the school nurse in George's care.

4. Discuss strategies for dealing with the power struggles George and his mother are having.

5. Do you think that George is a candidate for an insulin pump? Why or why not? Are there any ethical issues involved in your answer?

At this point, you have developed a basic understanding of diabetes in the school-age child. This understanding includes changing needs that occur with growth and development. Proceed to the next lesson for more on the application of teaching-learning principles in managing the problems of diabetes.

20

Teaching Self-Care to a Child with Diabetes and His Family

📖 **Reading Assignment:** Read about diabetes, focusing on aspects related to teaching and learning (Chapter 51, pages 1466-1483).

Patient: George Gonzalez, Room 301

Goal: Demonstrate application of teaching-learning principles for meeting the learning needs of a child with diabetes and his family.

Objectives:

- Identify learning needs of a child newly diagnosed with diabetes.
- Develop a sequential plan for teaching a child independence with care of diabetes.
- Discuss approaches to teaching various information and skills based on level of growth and development.
- Explore need for information, readiness, capability, and motivation as significant factors in the teaching-learning process.
- Differentiate roles of the child and the parent in managing the child's diabetes.

In this lesson, you will be focusing on the teaching aspect in the care of the child with diabetes. You will consider learning needs according to developmental stage and parental responsibilities, along with the dynamic nature of supervision and self-care.

You may need to review developmental issues associated with various age groups. You may also need to review the teaching-learning process since you will be applying principles throughout your work. You will assess needs, capabilities, readiness, and motivation. As you plan care, you will move beyond "teach about . . ." interventions and will begin more carefully articulating the content and method to be used. Content refers to the information or skill being taught. Method refers to the "how" of teaching. Explanation, role playing, and demonstration are just a few examples of methods.

Exercise 1

Clinical Preparation: Writing Activity

20 minutes

1. Review page 1473 in your text. How will you determine the learning needs of a child with diabetes and his family? What are your general thoughts about the influence of different developmental stages? (*Hint:* You do not need to break it down into age groups.) What is the role and responsibility of the family in care?

2. What if the child with diabetes is a toddler? What are some care issues? What might you suggest to parents?

3. What are some care issues if the child with diabetes is a preschooler? What might you suggest to parents?

4. Consider the needs of a school-age child with diabetes. What are some care issues? What might you suggest to parents?

5. What are some care issues if the child with diabetes is an adolescent? What might you suggest to parents?

6. You are teaching a family. Discuss areas of content that you would want to include about diabetes in general.

7. Did you consider the "honeymoon phase" as part of your discussion? Why is this significant to parent teaching? What should you say about it?

8. Explain how you would characterize the relationship among food, exercise, and insulin.

Exercise 2

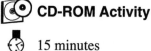 **CD-ROM Activity**

15 minutes

- Sign in to work at Pacific View Regional Hospital on the Pediatrics Floor for Period of Care 1. (*Note:* If you are already in the virtual hospital from a previous exercise, click on **Leave the Floor** and then **Restart the Program** to get to the sign-in window.)
- From the Patient List, select George Gonzalez.
- Click on **Go to Nurses' Station** and then on **301**.
- Click on **Patient Care** and then on **Nurse-Client Interactions**.
- Select and view the video titled **0730: Supervision—Glucose Testing**. (*Note:* If this video is not available, check the virtual clock to see whether enough time has elapsed. The video cannot be viewed before its specified time.)

1. Is George physically capable of being responsible for his own blood glucose testing?

2. What are some reasons why George may be noncompliant with blood glucose testing?

3. What does the nurse do that is effective? What other interventions can be offered?

4. Explain the content and methods you would use in teaching the skill of self administration of insulin.

5. What are possible barriers to learning the skill of injection technique?

6. List areas of content associated with discussing site rotations.

7. What is the site from which insulin is most rapidly absorbed?

8. Be creative. Develop a strategy for assisting with site rotations.

Exercise 3

 CD-ROM Activity

20 minutes

- Sign in to work at Pacific View Regional Hospital on the Pediatrics Floor for Period of Care 2. (*Note:* If you are already in the virtual hospital from a previous exercise, click on **Leave the Floor** and then **Restart the Program** to get to the sign-in window.)
- From the Patient List, select George Gonzalez.
- Click on **Go to Nurses' Station** and then on **301**.
- Click on **Patient Care** and then on **Nurse-Client Interactions**.
- Select and view the video titled **1115: Teaching—Disease Process**. (*Note:* If this video is not available, check the virtual clock to see whether enough time has elapsed. The video cannot be viewed before its specified time.)

1. Evaluate George's understanding of his condition and management of hypoglycemia.

2. What is his mother's level of understanding?

3. Given the responses of George and his mother, is there a need for teaching in this area? If so, what?

➤ • Click on **Leave the Floor** and then on **Restart the Program**.
  • Sign in to work at Pacific View Regional Hospital on the Pediatrics Floor for Period of Care 3.
  • From the Patient List, select George Gonzalez (Room 301).
  • Click on **Go to Nurses' Station**.
  • Click on Room **301**.
  • Click on **Patient Care**.
  • Click on **Nurse-Client Interactions**.
  • Select and view the video titled **1500: Teaching—Diabetic Diet**.

4. What is George's diet order? What are the recommendations of the dietitian?

5. What is the current thinking as to dietary recommendations for the child with diabetes?

6. Evaluate the nurse's teaching with regard to diet. What did she do well? What could have been better?

7. Discuss the effects of physical activity on blood sugar. Consider times of day when George might have more activity than others. What should he do to prevent any activity-related problems?

8. Based on the potential complications discussed in question 7, do you think George would be better not exercising? Explain your response. (*Hint:* Be sure to consider growth and development as a factor.)

Exercise 4

Clinical Preparation: Writing Activity

10 minutes

1. Health maintenance and regular visits with health care providers are important, even when the child is doing well. Discuss the issue of who (parent, child, or both) should be in attendance at an office visit.

2. What barriers do you see to providing optimal outpatient care for the child with diabetes and the family?

3. Discuss the advantages of diabetes groups or camps for a child like George.

Caring for a Teen with an Eating Disorder

👓 **Reading Assignment:** Read about eating disorders: Chapter 53 (pages 1539-1542).

Patient: Tiffany Sheldon, Room 305

Goal: Demonstrate an understanding of multidisciplinary care for a teenager with an eating disorder.

Objectives:

- Compare and contrast description, etiology, and typical behaviors associated with anorexia nervosa and bulimia nervosa.
- Discuss the physiologic impact of anorexia nervosa and bulimia nervosa.
- Discuss the multidisciplinary approach necessary for treatment of eating disorders.
- Explore the challenges of providing nursing care for clients with anorexia nervosa or bulimia nervosa.

In this lesson, you will explore a variety of challenges associated with caring for a teen with an eating disorder. You will care for Tiffany Sheldon, a 14-year-old with a history of 18 admissions within the past year for complications associated with anorexia nervosa. You will learn that helping a patient manage an eating disorder requires intensive multidisciplinary effort.

Exercise 1

 Clinical Preparation: Writing Activity

15 minutes

1. Compare and contrast anorexia and bulimia by matching each problem with its characteristics. (*Hint:* Although some behaviors may seem to overlap, they are usually associated more closely with one problem rather than the other. Choose the problem *most* closely associated with each characteristic.)

Characteristics	**Problem**
_____ Deliberate refusal of food to maintain body weight	a. Anorexia nervosa
_____ Recurrent episodes of binging and a sense of loss of control	b. Bulimia nervosa
_____ Excessive use of vomiting, laxatives, diuretics, or exercise	
_____ Possible amenorrhea—both primary and secondary	
_____ Overconcern with body image, though not distorted	
_____ Body image that is contrary to reality	
_____ Ritualistic eating pattern	
_____ Binge eating and purging	
_____ Muscle wasting, dull and brittle hair, lanugo	
_____ Risk for fluid and electrolyte imbalance	
_____ Tooth erosion	

2. Give an example of an eating pattern that might be found in a person with anorexia nervosa. What often underlies such behavior?

3. How is it believed that family function and culture play into the problem of eating disorders?

4. What are some secondary gains achieved through eating disorders? (*Hint:* Secondary gains are other benefits that the patient gets from his or her disease.)

Exercise 2

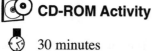 **CD-ROM Activity**

30 minutes

- Sign in to work at Pacific View Regional Hospital on the Pediatrics Floor for Period of Care 1. (*Note:* If you are already in the virtual hospital from a previous exercise, click on **Leave the Floor** and then **Restart the Program** to get to the sign-in window.)
- From the Patient List, select Tiffany Sheldon.
- Click on **Go to Nurses' Station**.
- Click on **Chart** and then on **305**.
- Review the **Nursing Admission** and the **History and Physical**.

1. What in Tiffany's history is indicative of her diagnosis of anorexia nervosa?

2. Did you identify the family crisis (divorce of parents) as a precipitating factor in Tiffany's situation? Did you include the fact that she is an "A" student in your list? Why should you see these factors as red flags?

• Click on **Return to Nurses' Station**.
• Click on Room **305** at the bottom of the screen.
• Click on **Patient Care**.
• Complete a head-to-toe assessment, watching for assessment data that are consistent with anorexia nervosa.

3. As you complete your assessment, what stands out for you? The patient's physical appearance? The systemic problems? How much does nutritional status affect the total patient?

→ • Click on **Nurse-Client Interactions**.

• Select and view the video titled **0730: Initial Assessment**. (*Note:* If this video is not available, check the virtual clock to see whether enough time has elapsed. The video cannot be viewed before its specified time.)

4. Tiffany has been described as having a flat affect, being withdrawn, and avoiding eye contact. How would you describe her behavior at the time of this interaction?

5. What is the most effective communication to use with Tiffany?

6. In addition to nursing assessment, what multidimensional assessments and interventions are important to developing an appropriate plan of care for Tiffany?

7. How do you think Tiffany might respond to being told that she will be seen by an Eating Disorders Team?

8. What is the nurse's role in identifying and/or coordinating care and services that Tiffany requires during her inpatient stay?

Exercise 3

 CD-ROM Activity

45 minutes

The first order of business with a patient who has anorexia nervosa is to correct any imbalances. Keep this in mind as you work through this exercise.

- Sign in to work at Pacific View Regional Hospital on the Pediatrics Floor for Period of Care 1. (*Note:* If you are already in the virtual hospital from a previous exercise, click on **Leave the Floor** and then **Restart the Program** to get to the sign-in window.)
- From the Patient List, select Tiffany Sheldon.
- Click on **Go to Nurses' Station**.
- Click on **Chart** and then on **305**.
- Review the chart, especially the **Physician's Orders** and the **Laboratory Reports**.

1. What is being done to assess for and manage Tiffany's fluid and electrolyte imbalance?

2. What do Tiffany's lab results tell you about her fluid and electrolyte status? Report on the ones that give you specific information.

3. Tiffany did not have a pH level done. A patient with anorexia nervosa is at risk for metabolic acidosis. What would happen to the pH in this instance?

4. List the objective assessment data that indicate Tiffany is dehydrated.

5. Why is Tiffany on a cardiac monitor?

6. Tiffany is receiving IV fluid with potassium chloride added. What is the order? What are the nursing responsibilities before and during potassium administration?

7. a. Identify a generic nursing diagnosis for hydration problems in patients with anorexia nervosa.

   b. Now rewrite this nursing diagnosis so that it accurately reflects Tiffany's situation.

Next, begin thinking about how adequate caloric intake is achieved.

→ • Click on **Return to Nurse's Station** and then on **Leave the Floor**.
  • From the Floor Menu, select **Restart the Program**.
  • Sign in to work at Pacific View Regional Hospital on the Pediatrics Floor for Period of Care 2.
  • From the Patient List, select Tiffany Sheldon.
  • Click on **Go to Nurses' Station** and then on Room **305** at the bottom of the screen.
  • Click on **Patient Care** and then on **Nurse-Client Interactions**.
  • Select and view the video titled **1115: Managing Anorexia Nervosa**.

8. Discuss the cultural beliefs and personal perceptions that influence the development of eating disorders. Consider both males and females in your discussion.

9. What is the value of an eating contract for Tiffany?

10. What is the rationale for the diet orders that are part of the eating contract?

11. Calculate Tiffany's daily caloric needs.

12. What supportive interventions might the nurse provide to help Tiffany remain compliant?

Now, consider the emotional aspects of Tiffany's care.

→ • Click on **Leave the Floor** and then **Restart the Program**.
  • Sign in to work at Pacific View Regional Hospital on the Pediatrics Floor for Period of Care 3.
  • From the Patient List, select Tiffany Sheldon.
  • Click on **Go to Nurses' Station**.
  • Click on Room **305** at the bottom of the screen.
  • Click on **Patient Care** and then on **Nurse-Client Interactions**.
  • Select and view the video titled **1500: Relapse—Contributing Factors**.

13. What does Tiffany say about what has caused her relapse? What recent events, if any, may have contributed to Tiffany having an acute episode of her anorexia nervosa?

14. What did the psychiatrist do to effectively elicit Tiffany's concerns?

15. What multidimensional factors will contribute to Tiffany's ability to comply with the eating contract that has been developed? What barriers may be present?

16. A patient with an eating disorder may not like the sensations associated with refeeding. Develop strategies to help Tiffany overcome barriers to the success of her eating disorder plan.

Exercise 4

Clinical Preparation: Writing Activity

15 minutes

1. Let's assume that Tiffany refuses to eat and her condition puts her at greater health risk. The hospital is awaiting a court order for a feeding tube. Tiffany will need to be restrained if the order is implemented. How will you handle this situation? What are your responsibilities as a nurse?

2. School nurses or nurses in community settings may play several roles with teens who have anorexia nervosa. Discuss one of the primary roles.

3. If you were a school nurse and a teen said to you, "I have to tell you something, but you can't tell anyone," how would you respond? What would your responsibilities be?

Generally, when the facilities are available, patients with eating disorders are transferred to an Eating Disorders Unit, where professionals are highly skilled and experienced with this area of care. However, this may not be the case in all settings; thus all nurses need to be aware of the problems, the risks, and the usual approaches to treatment. You have accomplished this by completing this lesson.

22

Caring for a Child and Family in the Emergency Department

Reading Assignment: Read about emergency care: Chapter 34 (pages 852-870).
Read about head injury: Chapter 52 (1496-1497, 1512-1515).

Patient: Tommy Douglas, Pediatrics Floor, Room 302

Goal: Demonstrate an appreciation of the needs and care for a child and family experiencing an emergency.

Objectives:

- Identify factors that may culminate in a stressful environment in the emergency department.
- Discuss nursing interventions supportive to the child and family who are in the emergency department.
- Discuss the concept of "across the room" assessment and priority setting for a child in the emergency department.
- Explore the implications of growth and development in emergency care.
- Explore medications frequently used in traumatic emergency situations.
- Identify priority concerns related to head injury.

In this lesson, you will explore the role of the nurse in emergency department care. More often than not, the priority needs of the child will be physiologic, but the psychosocial element of care cannot be ignored. Parents have many support needs that sometimes are pushed aside during the acute phase of the visit. You will learn general strategies for dealing with such issues. You will be working with 6-year-old Tommy Douglas, who has arrived in the emergency department after a blunt trauma injury.

Exercise 1

 Clinical Preparation: Writing Activity

20 minutes

1. List and explain five or six factors that can contribute to creating a stressful environment when a child is brought to the emergency department after a traumatic event.

2. For each of the factors you listed above, develop a nursing intervention to minimize stress. If you have had experience in such an environment (even during an observation), you have an opportunity to be creative here.

3. Review the general guidelines covered on page 853 of your textbook. How many of them did you incorporate in your intervention list? For any interventions you listed that are not in the textbook, consider how easy or realistic they would be to implement. Write a reflective comment.

4. What is the priority assessment on a new admission?

5. What is meant by the notion of "assessment from across the room"? Identify some assessments that can be made in this manner.

6. Rank the following care items in order of priority by numbering from 1 (highest priority) to 7 (lowest priority).

_____ Trauma scoring

_____ Assessment of child's coping

_____ Circulatory assessment

_____ History of injury

_____ Breathing assessment

_____ Airway assessment

_____ Signs of other injury

7. Choose two age groups of children that you would find especially challenging to work with in the emergency department. For each age group, explain the challenges and share a nursing intervention to help.

Parents and caregivers need a great deal of support. Nurses need to be able to anticipate fears and anxieties in crafting careful communication to elicit and respond to concerns.

8. What are the three greatest fears parents have when their child is brought to the emergency department?

9. Parents may feel pushed aside in the emergency department. How can the nurse deal with this problem?

Exercise 2

 CD-ROM Activity

45 minutes

- Sign in to work at Pacific View Regional Hospital on the Pediatrics Floor for Period of Care 1. (*Note:* If you are already in the virtual hospital from a previous exercise, click on **Leave the Floor** and then **Restart the Program** to get to the sign-in window.)
- From the Patient List, select Tommy Douglas.
- Click on **Go to Nurses' Station**.
- Click on **Chart** and then on **302**.
- Review Tommy's chart, especially the **Emergency Department** and **Physician's Orders** sections.

1. Review the circumstances of Tommy's admission. Include such information as the nature of his injury and the people around him.

2. Tommy reportedly fell from a swing and hit his head on concrete. This is considered to be a blunt trauma injury. Explain what is meant by blunt trauma.

3. Explain the mechanism of the acceleration-deceleration injury that occurs with a major head injury.

4. What are the priorities for initial management of a head injury?

5. A child with a head injury is at risk for _____ and

   _____.

6. List the signs of increased intracranial pressure.

7. Review Tommy's initial medication orders (from admission on Tuesday through Wednesday morning). List the medications ordered and give a reason for each order.

→ • Click on **Return to Nurses' Station**.
 • Click on the **Drug** icon in the lower left corner of the screen.
 • Review the medications ordered for Tommy, looking for any information you need to administer them.

8. Do you see any concerns? Explain.

Select one of the medications that needs to be administered during this period of care and complete the following steps to prepare and administer it.

→ • Click on **Return to Nurses' Station** and then on **Medication Room**.
 • Using the Five Rights, select, prepare, and administer the medication to be given. When you have finished the preparation, return to Tommy's room and administer the medication. (*Hint:* Although you should be getting more comfortable with the steps of preparing and administering medications, you can refer to pages 26-30 and 37-41 in the **Getting Started** section if you need help.)
 • To obtain feedback, click on **Leave the Floor**.
 • Click on **Look at Your Preceptor's Evaluations** and then on **Medication Scorecard**.

9. Review the feedback on your Medication Scorecard. Are there any areas in which you need to make changes? If so, select another medication ordered for Tommy and practice the procedure again.

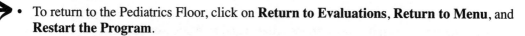

 • To return to the Pediatrics Floor, click on **Return to Evaluations**, **Return to Menu**, and **Restart the Program**.

• Sign in again to work with Tommy during Period of Care 1.

• Click on **Go to Nurses' Station**.

• Click on **Chart** and then on **302**.

• Click on **Physician's Orders**.

10. NaHCO$_3$ is ordered to be given STAT. How much time do you have to prepare and administer the medication?

11. Why is Tommy receiving bolus infusions?

 • Continue reviewing the Physician's Orders.

• Next, click on **Nursing Admission**.

12. The physician has ordered a rate increase for norepinephrine. At what rate was the drug running and to what rate has it been increased? (*Hint:* Find Tommy's weight in the Nursing Admission to do the necessary calculations.)

• Now click on the **Emergency Department** tab and search the record for neurologic assessment data.

13. What significant neurologic data did you find in Tommy's ED record?

14. Tommy is being stabilized in preparation for transfer to the Intensive Care Unit. A cerebral perfusion scan is done. What is the purpose of this test?

It is determined that Tommy will not be going to the Intensive Care Unit as planned. He is instead being transferred to the Pediatric Unit for end-of-life care.

→ • Click on **Return to Nurses' Station**.
 • Click on Room **302** at the bottom of the screen.
 • Click on **Patient Care**.
 • Complete a focused neurologic assessment of Tommy and then chart your findings in the EPR. (*Hint:* If you need help entering data in the EPR, refer to pages 15-16 in the **Getting Started** section of this workbook.)
 • To obtain feedback, click on **Leave the Floor** and then on **Look at Your Preceptor's Evaluations**.
 • Select **Examination Report** and review your evaluation.

15. Reflect on the completeness of your focused assessment of Tommy's neurologic status.

➜ • To return to the Pediatrics Floor, click on **Return to Evaluations**, **Return to Menu**, and **Restart the Program**.
   • Sign in again to work with Tommy for Period of Care 1.
   • Click on **Go to Nurses' Station**.
   • Click on **302** to go to Tommy's room.
   • Click on **Patient Care** and then on **Nurse-Client Interactions**.
   • Select and view the video titled **0730: Assessment—Neurological**.

16. Describe the Glasgow Coma Scale (GCS). Include the parameters that are assessed when it is used, particularly for children. (*Hint:* Review adaptations for children on page 1497 of your text.)

17. What was Tommy's GCS score?

18. Reflect on how well the nurse explained the use and meaning of the GCS. Do you think the parents found support during this interaction? What, if anything, would you have done differently?

➜ • Now select and view the video titled **0745: Intervention—Airway**. (*Note:* If this video is not available, check the virtual clock to see whether enough time has elapsed. The video cannot be viewed before its specified time.)

19. Tommy is using a ventilator. What is a ventilator used for? How would you expect Tommy's ventilator to be set?

20. How would you explain to Tommy's parents what the ventilator is doing?

21. Tommy's blood pressure is low. Explain why fluids help to maintain blood pressure.

Tommy will be receiving end-of-life care. Continue to the next lesson to learn about effective nursing care for the parents and family of a child who is dying.

Providing Support for Families Experiencing the Loss of a Child

👓 **Reading Assignment:** Read about care of the terminally ill: Chapter 36 (pages 920-929).

Read about ethical issues: Chapter 1 (pages 11-12).

Patient: Tommy Douglas, Room 302

Goal: Demonstrate an understanding of end-of-life care issues in the hospital setting.

Objectives:

• Explore the range of reactions that may occur when a family is told there is no hope of saving the child's life.
• Discuss the role of hospital ethics committees.
• Discuss nursing responsibilities associated with organ donation.
• Discuss the concept of "allowing" a child to die.
• Identify strategies to support parents and children as a child dies.

In this lesson, you will explore circumstances that may occur in hospital settings around a traumatic event resulting in certainty of death. Care for parents and other family members is the major focus during this time of hospice care. You will continue to work with the family of 6-year-old Tommy Douglas as he dies.

Exercise 1

💿 **CD-ROM Activity**

⏱ 30 minutes

• Sign in to work at Pacific View Regional Hospital on the Pediatrics Floor for Period of Care 2. (*Note:* If you are already in the virtual hospital from a previous exercise, click on **Leave the Floor** and then **Restart the Program** to get to the sign-in window.)
• From the Patient List, select Tommy Douglas.
• Click on **Go to Nurses' Station**.
• Click on Room **302** at the bottom of the screen.
• Click on **Patient Care** and then on **Nurse-Client Interactions**.

- Select and view the video titled **1115: The Family (Care) Conference**. (*Note:* If this video is not available, check the virtual clock to see whether enough time has elapsed. The video cannot be viewed before its specified time.)

1. Tommy has been certified as "brain dead" and a family conference has been held to inform Tommy's parents that he will not be helped by further intervention. Who are the usual participants in such a conference? What does each person bring to the discussion?

2. What is the role of the institutional ethics committee with respect to any potential conflicts in care delivery?

3. What intervention can the nurse provide to the parents after the family conference?

4. Assume that Tommy's family wants him to live "at all costs" and that they believe the parents of Terry Schiavo were correct in resisting removal of her feeding tube. How would you feel about this? What might be your response to Tommy's parents?

5. As Tommy's parents agree to organ donation, is there evidence of progression with anticipatory grieving?

6. Visit the website for United Network for Organ Sharing (*www.unos.org*). Discuss the criteria for donation and management of a potential donor.

→ • Click on **Chart** and then on **302**.
  • Click on **Physician's Orders** and review.

7. Discuss the kind of care that is being provided for Tommy during this time.

8. Tommy is receiving hospice care. Contrast palliative and hospice care.

Let's check in on Tommy's family a little later in the day.

→ • Click on **Leave the Floor** and then on **Restart the Program**.
   • Sign in to care for Tommy Douglas, this time during Period of Care 3.
   • Click on **Go to Nurses' Station** and then on Room **302** at the bottom of the screen.
   • Click on **Patient Care**.
   • Click on **Nurse-Client Interactions**.
   • Select and view the video titled **1500: Nurse-Family Communication**.

9. Evaluate the nurse's approach in dealing with a family in crisis. Did the nurse demonstrate empathy? If so, how?

10. Is the nurse's body language congruent with his verbal communication?

11. Present an alternative to the nurse's approach if you believe it is indicated.

Exercise 2

Clinical Preparation: Writing Activity

30 minutes

"Allowing" a child to die is a very difficult concept. Parents go through several stages as their child dies.

1. Discuss what parents go through when their child experiences a life-threatening injury or illness that then becomes terminal.

2. Parents frequently need to talk about what is happening while their child is dying. Why?

3. What anticipatory guidance would you offer parents for dealing with other children in their family?

4. What information needs to be provided about the dying process?

5. How might you guide parents at the time of death? (*Hint:* Remember that allowing a child to die is tremendously difficult for parents.)

6. How are siblings of a dying child likely to view death?

7. How would you provide care for the family members after their child's death?

8. Assume that you enter the room and find the parents sobbing as they sit with their dying child. Does this mean you have not been effective with your teaching and care? What can you do for these parents?

9. What do you think the concept of "chronic sorrow" means?

10. How do you think you might react to caring for a dying child and the family? Do you think you could be effective? Explain your response.

11. Discuss ways that nurses who care for dying children cope with their own grief.

You have had the opportunity to consider care of the terminally ill child and many of the issues that might arise. This experience will help you to be more effective with your nursing care in similar situations—and it will help you take better care of yourself.